Mind Control Master:
Toxoplasma's Life Cycle

Shiva

Table of contents

3. Introduction

3.1 *Toxoplasma gondii*

3.1.1 General introduction

Toxoplasma gondii is an ubiquitous apicomplexan parasite first discovered in 1908 by Charles Nicolle in Tunisia in the native rodent *Ctenodactylus gundi* (1). *T. gondii* is generally transmitted by the fecal-oral route and has a heteroxenous life cycle described in Fig. 1a. Sexual replication takes place in the intestinal tracts of felids, definitive hosts for the parasite, and leads to the dissemination in the environment of infectious oocysts. When oocysts are ingested by any non-felid warm-blooded mammal, the asexual expansion phase of the parasite happens. Actively replicating tachyzoites disseminate through the host system and, upon immune pressure, convert into a slowly replicative phase as bradyzoites. The latter form tissue cysts within skeletal muscles and the central nervous system and they are believed to persist throughout the whole host life (2). One of the reasons for *T. gondii*'s great success resides in the capability of horizontal infection between different intermediate hosts, e.g. from infected pigs to humans, since not only the oocyst form of the parasite is infectious, but the tissue residing bradyzoite form as well. This peculiarity allows the parasite to bypass the sexual phase of the cycle and is to date a unique characteristic within Apicomplexa (3). Therefore *T. gondii* can be acquired via food and toxoplasmosis is considered a zoonotic disease. It is estimated that one third of the world human population is currently infected with *T. gondii* (4), but country-specific diets or hygienic conditions might lead to even higher numbers. For examples, a recent study in Germany reported that half of the population is positive for anti-*T. gondii* antibodies, with a 24 % difference in prevalence between the former East and West of the country, likely due to different dietary habits (5) .

Being part of the phylum *Apicomplexa*, *T. gondii* is characterized by the presence of the apical complex structure which mediates invasion, and of the apicoplast, a four membrane-bound organelle which is a residual of an endosymbiotic algae (3). The parasite has an obligate intracellular lifestyle and, during an active invasive process, forms a parasitophorous vacuole membrane (PVM) consisting of both host and parasite proteins. Indeed, during invasion *T. gondii* secretes numerous proteins in a time-controlled and regulated process from several secretory organelles (represented in Fig. 1b). First, micronemes secrete microneme proteins (MIC) which are essential for attachment to and invasion of the host cell. Subsequently, the elongated rhoptry organelles discharge rhoptry neck and bulb proteins, RON and ROP respectively, which are involved in invasion as well as mediating the first parasite defense towards host immune responses. The role of specific ROPs is further discussed in section 3.3.3. Finally, numerous dense granule proteins (GRA) are secreted in two distinct releases by the dense granule organelles and are crucial for host immune-modulation (reviewed in (6)). Altogether, these conserved groups of proteins highlight the parasitic ductile nature of *T. gondii* and provide evidence for the parasite replicative success in different host and cell types.

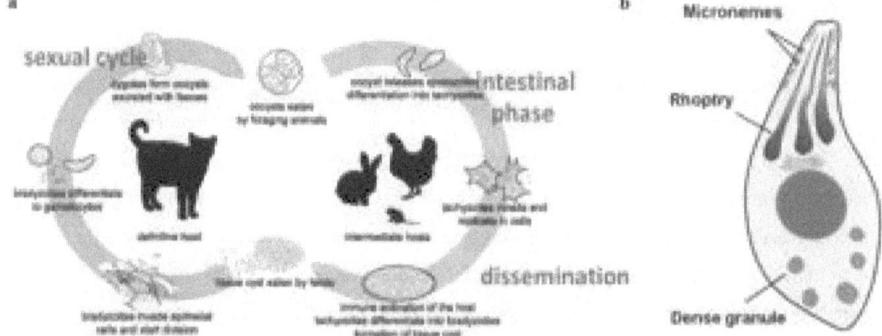

Fig 1. Life cycle of *T. gondii* and structure of the tachyzoite form of the parasite. (a) The heteroxenous life cycle of *T. gondii* includes both a sexual phase in felids and an asexual stage in intermediate hosts. Image from Lilue et al. (7) **(b)** Schematic representation of *T. gondii* secretory organelles during the tachyzoite form of the parasite. Image from English et al. (8)

3.1.2   *T. gondii* genotypes

The global population of *T. gondii* can be divided into three main clonal lineages, named type I, II and III, and a more recently identified type 12 (9-11). Type II and 12 are the most common lineages found in Europe and North America, followed by type III (12). On the contrary, type I is rare in these areas and more frequently found in Asia (13). In the last years a more detailed genotyping based on 11 loci led to the re-classification into 15 haplogroups within 6 major clades (14). To date 231 *T. gondii* genotypes have been identified based on Polymerase Chain Reaction - Restriction Fragment Length Polymorphysm (PCR-RFLP) analysis (source: ToxoDB, (15)). With this new classification a multitude of atypical isolates with haplotypes different from previously defined strains were identified, mostly in South America. Analogous diversity has also been observed with a microsatellite genotyping-based approach (16).

Even though less frequent, atypical and mixed genotypes have been also found in Europe. *T. gondii* type I alleles were already identified in European human cases in the initial study by Howe and Sibley (9). With the new reached consensus about genotyping criteria (17), knowledge about genotypes present in Europe is currently expanding, unveiling a diversity higher than expected. Type I and atypical genotypes were identified in domestic cats in Germany (18), farm animals from Portugal and Austria (19) as well as in human samples in Denmark (20). Surprisingly, a recent extensive screening of raw meat products in Poland found clonal type I and mixed genotypes in 10 % and 23 % of the *T. gondii*-positive samples respectively (21). These evidences highlight that, apart from the widespread clonal type II, other virulent clonal strains as well as atypical genotypes have been identified in Europe in human and domestic animals alike.

3.1.3 ROP-mediated virulence of *T. gondii* genotypes

Genotyping of strains is not only useful for classification purposes, but a correlation between parasite strains and virulence exists (22). *T. gondii* virulence has been defined in laboratory *Mus musculus* with type I being the most virulent clonal lineage. Different outcomes have been identified according to the way of infection –i.e. intraperitoneal, oral, subcutaneous and intranasal– and the parasite stage; however the most common approach and the one suggested as gold standard is intraperitoneal injection of tachyzoites (23). Further research is required to understand the reason underneath these differences and their impact on the current strains classification. All type I strains have a lethal effect on laboratory mice when tachyzoites are injected intraperitoneally, and host death occurs within 9 and 14 days post infection depending on specific parasite and mouse strains combinations (24). Type II and III have progressively less virulence (24).

Comparisons between virulent and avirulent *T. gondii* strains led to the identifications of the two key virulence factors: the rhoptry proteins ROP18 and ROP5 (25-28). The allelic combination of these two highly polymorphic genes is predictive on *T. gondii* virulence in mice (29) and ROP5 deletion in type I strains is sufficient to completely attenuate acute virulence. These two proteins act as complex with ROP17 to phosphorylate and inactivate proteins mediating the host innate response (30), via a mechanism further explained in section 3.3.3. The ROP family has the highest number of copy number variation (CNV) within the *T. gondii* genome and has an elevated frequency of nonsynonymous versus synonymous mutations (31). Diversity within the ROP gene family, as well as in the family of surface antigens protein (SAG) genes, is what mostly differentiates *T. gondii* strains. This highlights the importance of the ROP family for *T. gondii* and supports the hypothesis of important roles of these genes as pathogenesis determinants.

ROP virulent alleles are not only predictors of virulence for mice but also in human hosts (29). Indeed, type I strains are more frequently genotyped in symptomatic toxoplasmosis cases, such as ocular disease, congenital acquisition or reactivation of a chronic infection in immunocompromised patients (32). Humans lack the murine immune proteins specifically phosphorylated by the ROP triad, however novel targets of rhoptry proteins have been recently identified in human hosts. For example ROP18 phosphorylates the transcriptional factor ATF6β resulting in a decreased antigen presentation in CD8[+] T cells (33). Further, a role for ROP18 in the development of *T. gondii*-related encephalitis have been recently unveiled (34). Therefore a deeper understanding of virulent parasite strains distribution and identification of their natural reservoir has a major clinical importance.

3.2 Reservoir of virulent *T. gondii* strains

3.2.1 Dietary habits of cats

T. gondii parasites persist in nature only if they reach the definitive hosts and are shed in form of infectious oocysts. Infection via environmental contamination and vertical transmission are thought to occur rarely in Felidae (3, 35). On the contrary, the main infection route in cats is represented by ingestion of infective bradyzoite cysts from intermediate hosts. Interestingly this stage is also the most infective one for felids, suggesting how *T. gondii* evolved to support the main infection route (36). Recently, oocysts shedding from adult seropositive cats following re-infection has been observed (37), which questions the dogma of the single shedding event in a cat lifetime. This implies that ingestion of each infected prey might contribute to *T. gondii* spread in the environment. Therefore looking at felids' preys could help us identifying important reservoir of *T. gondii* genotypes.

The variety of Felidae that populates Europe is lower than in other parts of the planet, and is mostly represented by the domestic cat (*Felis silvestris catus*) and to a lesser extent by the wild cat (*Felis silvestris silvestris*) and a hybrid population of the two. Given the higher number and ubiquitous presence of these felid species, especially the domestic cat, their major role in *T. gondii* oocysts dissemination is expected. Information regarding dietary habits of cats indicate that their diet is mainly composed of small mammals, of which Rodentia is the most preyed order (38, 39). Birds and lagomorphs (hares and rabbits), despite being universally reported, are less often preyed. Within the Rodentia order, one of the least preyed species is *Rattus* spp., likely because of their bigger size and less palatability, whereas other small rodents species constitute their major diet item (38). Therefore, the focus of this book is on the most represented small rodent species and data from different studies in Europe are collected in Table 1.

It is evident that European felids prey more on rodents of the family Cricetidae, e.g. the Arvicolinae bank vole *Myodes glareolus* (formerly *Clethrionomys glareolus*) and *Microtus* spp. –both referred as "voles" in the rest of the work–, or the Muridae *Apodemus* spp., rather than *Mus musculus* species –the latter named "mice"–. Despite variation in prey availability is known to cause changes in felids' diet (38) which thus implies geographical differences, *Apodemus* spp. and *Microtus* spp. are overall the preferred preys. A comprehensive and recent review on dietary habits of European felids, confirms the mentioned non-murine rodent species being more preyed than *Mus* spp. (40). Most of the studies are based on morphological examination of feline stomach and gut content or scats, and less often based on preys brought home as trophies, the latter being less reliable since they do not imply ingestion. Of note is the study of Forin-Wiart et al. where for the first time metabarcoding of cat feces to determine prey composition was used (41). Overall, data are in accordance confirming that in Europe *M. glareolus*, *Microtus* spp. and *Apodemus* spp. are more often preyed than *Mus spp.*

Table 1. Prey items of European domestic, wild and hybrid cats. D = Domestic cats: W = Wild cats; H = Hybrid cats.

Reference	Location	Cats	Preyed species [%]			
			Mus spp.	*Apodemus* spp.	*Microtus* spp.	*M. glareolus*
(42)	Hungary	D	7.0	13.8	37.7	9.6
		W	0.0	28.1	33.3	1.8
		H	1.6	9.4	25.0	18.8
(43)	France	D	8.0	4.0	16.0	0.0
		W	5.0	33.0	13.0	10.0
		H	3.0	17.0	14.0	8.0
(44)	Italy	W	0.2	64.9	11.2	12.2
(45)	Portugal	W	0.0	71.3	35.4	0.0
(46)	UK	D	4.3	11.4	9.8	3.8
(47)	Slovakia	W	0.0	9.4	72.9	10.4
(41)	France	D	0.2	1.3	27.3	2.7

These small rodent species are widespread in Europe with slightly different habitats. *Mus* spp. and in particular the house mouse, *M. musculus*, are found both in anthropized environments and agriculture and often considered as pests. The epidemic dispersion of the house mouse is thought as responsible for the domestication of cats (38). *Apodemus* spp. resemble the house mouse in terms of morphology and habitat, with slight differences according to the subspecies. Voles like *Microtus arvalis and Microtus agrestis* are smaller in size compared to *Muridae* and can be found in cities as well as in grassland, whereas *M. glareolus* prefers woodland (source: IUCN red list of threatened species and the mammal society (48)). The species above have a lifespan of one to two years, longer for voles than mice, mostly depending on the presence of predators. Due to the ubiquitous presence of cats in Europe, these rodent species and one of their major predators are sympatric. A recent study held in Berlin by Krucken et al. showed that indeed all mentioned species are present in the urban and suburban environment and are infected with *T. gondii* (49).

Voles as *M. glareolus* and *Microtus* spp. are reservoir of numerous zoonotic diseases as viruses like tick-borne encephalitis virus and cowpox virus, bacteria such as *Leptospira* spp., *Bartonella* spp., *Rickettsia* spp., *Borrelia* spp. and unicellular eukaryotic parasites like *Giardia* spp., *Cryptosporidium* spp. and *Babesia microti* (50-55). In the last years *M. glareolus* attracted increased attention for being the main host for Puumala orthohantavirus (PUUV) whom infection provokes increasing cases of hemorrhagic fever with renal syndrome (HFRS) in humans, occasionally with lethal outcome (56). However, studies focussing on these natural reservoirs are largely underrepresented. Nevertheless, non-murine rodents of the mentioned species are gaining increased interest in the field of wild- or eco-immunology because of their role as natural reservoirs and carriers of the genetic variability lost in inbred mouse colonies (57).

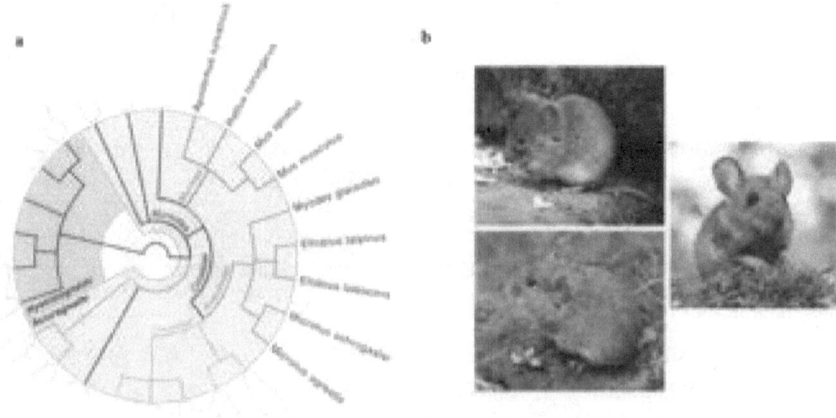

Fig. 2. Taxonomic tree of rodent species (a) A taxonomic species tree based on phylogenetic relationship between the rodent species mentioned in this work (tree computed at https://www.ncbi.nlm.nih.gov/Taxonomy/CommonTree/wwwcmt.cgi). Image as part of Fig. 4 from the published manuscript Ehret et al. (58) **(b)** From top left clockwise: *M. glareolus* (credits Roger Butterfield), *A. sylvaticus* and *M. agrestis* (credits Rudmer Zwerver).

3.2.2   *T. gondii* infection in European rodents

Another factor contributing to the likelihood of *T. gondii* genotypes maintenance in nature is the frequency of cat's preys infection. The prevalence of infection of most preyed species mentioned in the previous chapter ranges between 0.0 and 34.9 % in Europe (Table 2). Despite a general low prevalence of *T. gondii* in the considered species, data suggest that *M. glareolus*, *Microtus* spp. and *Apodemus* spp. are more often infected than *Mus* spp. Of notice are the high prevalence values for *M. musculus* and *Apodemus* spp. registered in UK. Authors of these studies found constant high prevalence in rodents at different ages, even in the absence of cats in the environment (59), and conserved genotypes in rodent populations (60, 61), suggesting high levels of vertical transmission.

It is crucial to consider that only rodents resistant to infection will be identified in these studies, since susceptible hosts will die of acute toxoplasmosis. Several studies indicate that not only different susceptibility to *T. gondii* exists within inbred laboratory mouse strains (23) and between different *Mus musculus* subspecies (7, 62), but also between different rodent species. For example a study performing *in vivo* infection of wild animals of all the mentioned rodent species with a fresh virulent clinical isolate concluded that these more preyed species are also more resistant to infection compared to *Mus* spp. (63).

In particular *M. glareolus* is by far the most resistant, followed by *Microtus arvalis* and *Apodemus flavicollis*, then *Microtus agrestis* and *Apodemus agrarius*. Importantly, and differently from other *in vivo* studies, *Mus* rodents were also trapped from the wild; therefore the result was not influenced by confounders linked to laboratory animal models (58). Furthermore, results were independent of the infection route of choice. In agreement with this study, *in vivo* experiments on *Microtus arvalis* (64) and corean *Apodemus agrarius* (65) confirmed their less susceptibility to virulent *T. gondii* than C57BL/6 inbred mice via all tested infection routes. Interestingly a fully genotyped isolate from naturally infected rodents reports the formation of virulent parasite brain cysts in a living vole, highlighting the resistance of the latter to infection and its potential as intermediate host (66, 67).

Taken together these data support the hypothesis that *M. glareolus*, *Microtus* spp. and *Apodemus* spp. might be reservoir of virulent *T. gondii*, given both their higher infection rate and their lower susceptibility to virulent parasite infection compared to *Mus* spp.

Table 2. ***T. gondii* infection in rodent species in Europe.** Na = not assessed. PCR = polymerase chain reaction; WB = Western Blot; SF = Sabin-Feldman dye test.

			Prevalence [%]			
Reference	**Location**	**Diagnostic method**	*Mus* spp.	*Apodemus* spp.	*Microtus* spp.	*M. glareolus*
(49)	Berlin (Germany)	PCR	na	4.3	31.0	0.0
(18)	Germany	PCR, WB	0.0	0.0	0.0	0.0
(68)	Czech Republic	SF	0.7	8.3	3.5	1.0
(69)	France and Portugal	SF	0.7	0.8	0.0	0.0
(70)	Netherlands	PCR	9.0	0.0	4.2	0.0
(61)	UK	PCR	na	34.9	na	na
(71)	UK	SF	na	20.0	na	17.6
(59)	UK	PCR	59	na	na	na

3.3 Host immune response during *T. gondii* infection

Mechanisms of host immune responses during *T. gondii* infection have been widely studied in many host species. The initial phase of infection corresponds to the ingestion of infective oocysts or bradyzoites and their differentiation in actively dividing tachyzoites within the host intestine. This phase is still the least known stage and surely deserve to be more addressed in the near future (reviewed in (72)). The host response to tachyzoite infection is the most commonly studied and well-known stage. Conserved feature between different host species is the pivotal role of the IFN-γ cytokine. Indeed, mice deficient of IFN-γ or its receptor, or when the cytokine binding is blocked via antibody neutralization, display higher susceptibility to infection (73-75). Similarly, the cytokine promotes parasite clearance in human cells (76).

IFN-γ is secreted by natural killer (NK) cells first and CD4$^+$ and CD8$^+$ lymphocytes later, following stimulation with the interleukine 12 (IL-12) (reviewed by Hunter and Sibley (77)). Major triggers for IL-12 release from macrophages and dendritic cells differ between mice and humans. Murine phagocytic cells can directly recognize the main *T. gondii* antigen profilin via Toll-Like Receptors (TLR) 11 and 12, as well as phagocytise infected cells or opsonized parasites. Human cells rely on the latter mechanisms, since they do not have functional TLR11 and TLR12. Only recently, a novel mechanism of human immune response mediated by the release of an alarmin from infected cells was identified (78). In both human and murine cells, IFN-γ pathway activation induces several mechanisms to promote parasite clearance, like production of reactive oxygen species (ROS) and nitric oxyde (NO). Humans have IFN-γ-mediated control mechanisms of *T. gondii* infection that have not been identified in the mouse model so far, e.g. limitation of iron and tryptophane supply and induction of an inflammasome-mediated death (77). The main resistance mechanism in mice, mediated by the Immunity Related GTPase family of proteins (IRG, further discussed in section 3.3.3) is also unique of this host family and induced by IFN-γ.

3.3.1 The IFN-γ pathway

IFN-γ binds as a homodimer to its cell surface receptor –composed of subunits IFN-γR1 and IFN-γR2– leading to subsequent activation of the Janus Kinase (JAK)-mediated signal transduction pathway (79). Signal transducer and activator of transcription 1 (STAT1) is the main transcription factor that is activated by engagement of the IFN-γ receptor. Phosphorylation on tyrosine 701 (Tyr701) and serine 727 (Ser727) and subsequent dimerization of STAT1 leads to its nuclear translocation where it induces the expression of several target genes via binding to the γ-interferon-Activation Sites (GAS) and Interferon-Stimulated Response Elements (ISRE) in their promoter region (80, 81).

Following IFN-γ treatment more than 4,000 genes varying 2 folds or more have been identified in the mouse model to date, and more than the double in human cells (82). This cytokine's main function is to activate cellular immune responses to the invading pathogen, including bacteria, viruses and parasites. The two main families of proteins induced by IFN-γ treatment are Immunity-Related GTPases (IRG) and Guanylate Binding Proteins (GBP) (83), both part of the defense mechanism proper of each nucleated cell named cell-autonomous immunity (84). When a pathogen succeeds in invading the host cell, the cell-autonomous response represents the last line of defense against the pathogen. Indication of the importance of IFN-γ-regulated cell-autonomous genes is their expansion within genome clusters and tight regulation, both costly processes for the host cell. These two families of genes are broadly conserved between plants and vertebrate mammals and they are expressed in hematopoietic as well as non-hematopoietic cells (85).

The importance of the IFN-γ-mediated immune response in *T. gondii* infection is evident from the evolution of parasite mechanisms specifically inhibiting this cytokine pathway and the downstream transcriptional factor STAT1-mediated gene expression. The mechanism is conserved in all three clonal lineages and results in the transcriptional repression of almost half of the interferome (86). Interestingly the expression of crucial *Irg* genes like *Irga6* and *Irgb6* was reduced by at least 2-fold following infection with all the tested strains. Mediator of STAT1 transcriptional repression is TgIST (*T. gondii* inhibitor of STAT1 transcriptional activity), a protein secreted by the parasite into the host cytoplasm (87, 88). TgIST reaches the host nucleus where it sequesters the phosphorylated form of STAT1 in chromatin-bound repressor complexes (89). The blocked recycling of STAT1 leads to a decreased expression of IFN-γ-induced genes and confers the parasite a crucial advantage during infection (90). TgIST is just one example of the numerous parasite tools to alter host signalling and immune response, recently reviewed by Hakimi et al (32).

3.3.2 Immunity Related GTPases

Immunity Related GTPases are conserved in many vertebrate genomes but with species differences regarding copy number and chromosome loci. For example, they are present in fish but absent in birds, and within mammals present in dogs but not cats. Primates lost *IRGs* with the exception of *IRGC*, locally expressed in the testis, and *IRGM* (91, 92). Rodents have the biggest *Irg* diversity described so far, counting 23 *Irg* genes in C57BL/6 mice encoded in large gene clusters located on chromosomes 7, 11 and 18 ((91) Fig. 6b). Their tight regulation via IFN-γ is highlighted by the presence of GAS and ISRE elements in the promoter regions regulating their expression (91). IRGs play key roles in murine resistance against a wide variety of intracellular pathogens such as parasites like *Toxoplasma gondii*, bacteria as *Chlamydia trachomatis*, *Mycobacteria tubercolosis*, *Salmonella typhimurium* and *Listeria monocytogenes*, and fungi like the microsporidia *Encephalitozoon cuniculi* (93-99). IRGs seem also involved during bacterial infection in lower vertebrate (100).

IRGs are 21-47 kDa proteins that have been recently classified in three main categories based on their described functions: effector, regulatory and decoy IRGs ((7) Fig. 3).

Effector IRGs, as IRGa6 and IRGb6, are recruited on the PVM of invading pathogens and mediate its disruption via still unclear mechanisms. As GTPases they hydrolyze GTP which is paramount for protein dimerization and membrane loading (101). IRGa6 is the only crystalized protein of the family, and sequence comparison predicts that its structure well represents the IRG 47 kDa protein family (101).

Regulatory IRGs, as IrgM1-3 in mice and IRGM in humans, are necessary to regulate the activity of effector IRGs. Interestingly, large genome-wide association studies linked specific human *IRGM* alleles with the development of inflammatory disorders like Crohn's disease, possibly via a lack of IRGM-mediated regulation of the inflammasome assembly (102). Murine IRGm1 and IRGm3 localize at different intracellular organelles' membranes and display a regulatory function by keeping effector IRGs in a GDP-bound inactive state (103). IRGm3 is necessary for PVM disruption and for host resistance to avirulent strains infection (104), and mediates the PVM stripping and blebbing into the cytoplasm of murine astrocytes (105).

Decoy IRGs count at the moment only IRGb2-b1, whose activity is described thoroughly in section 3.3.4. However, *Irgb2-b1* gene structure, two single classic *Irg* exons separated by a long 6 kb intron and translated as 2.5 kb long mRNA, is analogous to other three genes, i.e. *Irgb5-b4*, *Irgb9-b8* and the pseudogene *Irgb5-b3*. Their function has not been documented yet, thus redundancy of decoy IRG cannot be excluded at the moment.

Overall it seems that, at least in the mouse model, the IRG system covers the role of powerful immune Swiss Army knife, with many functions identified and still mysterious tools to figure out.

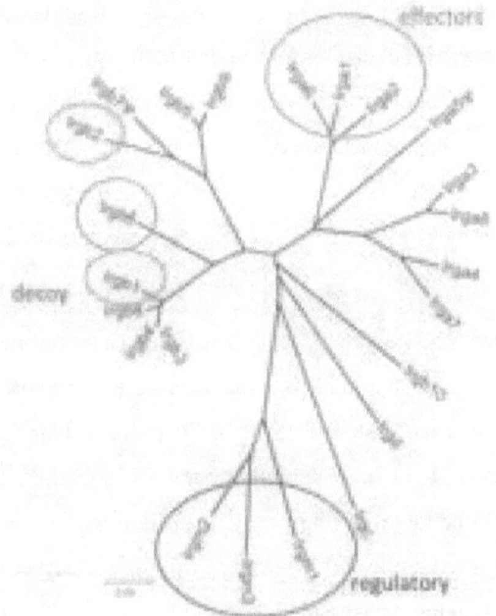

Fig. 3. Immunity Related GTPases (*Irgs*) of *M. musculus*. Unrooted tree (p-distance based on neighbour-joining method) of nucleotide sequences of the G-domains of the 23 Irg GTPases in the mouse BL6 genome (genome ID 52). Highligthed the three categories of *Irg* genes: regulatory, effector and decoy *Irgs*. The image was modified from Bekpen et al (91).

3.3.3 Effector IRG role during *T. gondii* infection

During *T. gondii* infection of IFN-γ-primed cells, effector IRGs like IRGa6 and IRGb6 are relocated from different organelles, as the endoplasmic reticulum and the Golgi apparatus respectively, on the parasite membrane in a GTP-dependent fashion observed both *in vitro* and *in vivo* (106, 107). These IRGs mediate vacuole rupture and are necessary to limit *T. gondii* avirulent growth. Effector IRG loading is hierarchical, with pioneers IRGb10 and IRGb6 followed by IRGa6 (108). Loading of parasite vacuoles starts as soon as few minutes after infection and increases progressively up to 2 hpi covering almost the totality of type II and III PVM, whereas type I parasite PVM are scarcely coated (108). First, loading of avirulent parasites' PVM results in morphological changes of the vacuole and the parasite within, both of them rounding up. Then, the parasitophorous vacuole membrane permeabilizes, followed by the parasite membrane itself few minutes later (105, 109). Given the change in shape of the vacuole, it has been hypothesized that the trigger for PVM rupture is the mechanical pressure caused by oligomerization of IRGs and GBPs. By electronic microscopy, it was observed that vacuole rupture happens by opening of the PVM and formation of vesicles which protrude in the host cytoplasm (105). IRGs display a dynamin-like phenotype despite the fact that they do not share sequence similarities and that their vesicle coating might regulate trafficking for intracellular degradation. Afterwards, GBP2 directly binds the plasma membrane of free intracellular parasites, likely contributing to its killing, recently showed by high-resolution live-cell imaging (110).

Following PVM rupture and along with the parasite killing, the cell starts a process of programmed cell death with features of pyronecrosis, meaning loss in cell membrane integrity and release of the pro-inflammatory chromatine remodelling protein HMBG1, observed both in murine macrophages and fibroblasts (109). Despite a not clear association of the autophagosome marker LC3 with the PVM (106) and no exposure of the autophagy-associated phosphatidyl serine on the plasma membrane (109), members of the autophagy pathway like Atg5 are necessary to mediate IRGs loading (108) and parasite killing (111).

This host mechanism protects only against infection with avirulent but not with virulent strains. As already anticipated in chapter 3.1.3, virulent parasites express ROP5 proteins (27, 28) which bind to IRGa6, and to a lesser extent to IRGb6 and IRGb10, to prevent their GTP-hydrolysis and protein oligomerization on the PVM (112, 113). ROP5 binding induces a conformational change that exposes IRGa6 Thr102 and Thr108 to be target of phosphorylation from ROP17 and ROP18 respectively (30, 114). Eventually, the synergistic activity of the virulent ROP triad succeeds in hijacking the host cell-autonomous response thus allowing parasite replication.

3.3.4 The role of IRGb2-b1 in mediating resistance to virulent *T. gondii*

Intraperitoneal injection of virulent *T. gondii* strains always have a lethal effect on inbred laboratory *M. musculus* strains (24). In 2013 Lilue et al. showed that the wild-derived *M. musculus castaneus* Indian strain CIM survives infection with the virulent GT1 strain whereas, as expected, all inbred NMRI mice die within 15 days (7). A genetic backcross between resistant and susceptible strains identified the *Irg* locus on chromosome 11 to be associated with the resistant phenotype. Interestingly, *Irg* genes are conserved in laboratory mice due to breeding, whereas high diversity was observed in wild-derived mice (7). Furthermore, cloning of one of the most diverse genes, the tandem *Irgb2-b1*$_{CIM}$, in susceptible fibroblasts resulted in the ROP5-mediated phosphorylation of the transfected protein instead of the key immune mediator IRGa6. Phosphorylation of Irga6 implies loss of function of the protein, therefore the "decoy" activity of IRGb2-b1 allows the host cell to still mount an IRG-mediated response to infection. Structural mimicry of IRGb2-b1 to IRGa6 is suggested by the fact that the first was crystalized as dimer and the latter is only found as tandem protein of subunits with the same size (101). CIM-derived *Irgb2-b1* KO cells lose their resistance to infection, supporting the hypothesis of a protective role of the protein during virulent *T. gondii* infection (115). More recently, it has been showed that resistance to virulent strain infection is not only dependant on the genetic variability of wild-derived mice, but is also linked to *M. musculus* subspecies (62). In particular, *M. musculus domesticus* shows susceptibility to infection regardless of inbred or outbred strain choice. On the contrary *M. musculus castaneus* strains, including the CIM strain already investigated by Lilue et al., as well as *M. musculus musculus* PWK/Ph strains are resistant to infection regardless of breeding. In agreement with the work of Lilue et al., resistance is associated with the region of chromosome 11 encompassing the *Irg* genes. This work further highlights the critical protective role of IRG proteins during *T. gondii* infection in a major host as *M. musculus*.

Phylogenetic analyses revealed positive pressure in rhoptry proteins' residues involved in binding to IRGs as well as in the target threonine on IRGa6 (30, 116). Furthermore, the whole region at the interface with ROP5 is under selective pressure and is enriched with nonsynonymous versus synonymous substitutions, both in *Irga6* and *Irgb2* genes (7, 116). This suggests co-evolution mechanisms between the *T. gondii* main virulence factor and the murine target IRGa6, resulting in virulent parasites success in infection. Similarly, IRGb2-b1 was suggested as the host response to virulent parasite evolution, which evolved only in certain host species. Overall the ROP5-IRG system is an example of the evolutionary arms race between the host immune responses and pathogen virulence (117). Analysis of further host species' *Irg* might lead to the identification of virulent parasites reservoirs, similarly to what described for *Mus* spp.

The *T. gondii* infection events described in the last sections are graphically shown in Fig. 4. The table includes both the host response to virulent and avirulent *T. gondii* in murine inbred cell systems, and the resistant molecular mechanism of *M. musculus castaneus* CIM cells.

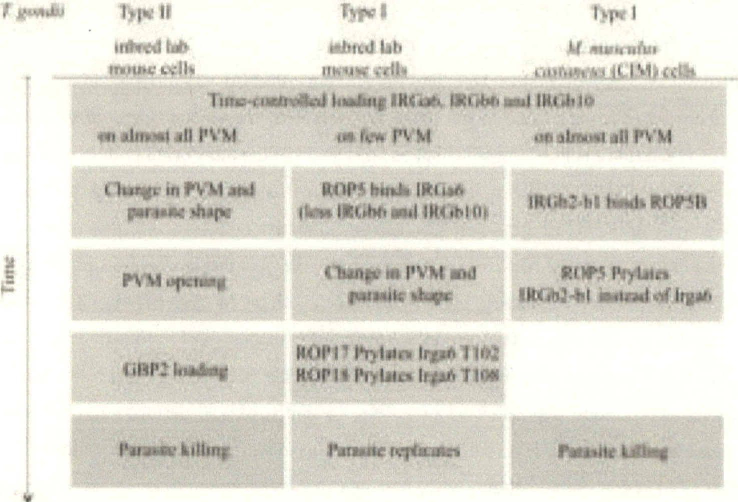

Fig. 4. Scheme of early events during in vitro *T. gondii* infection in inbred laboratory mice and wild-derived *M. musculus castaneus* (CIM). Data reported in the scheme are from the following studies (7, 30, 105, 108-110, 114-116). "Prylates" stands for phosphorylates.

3.4 Aims of the study

Rodents surely constitute a crucial intermediate host for *T. gondii*, because of their ubiquitous presence, their ability to develop chronic infections and their central role in the diet of the parasite's main definite host, the domestic cat. Most of the research on protozoan parasites is carried on in laboratory inbred *M. musculus*, and *T. gondii* is not an exception (58). All *T. gondii* strains require a suitable host that is tolerant to infection and develops chronic infection in order to reach the definitive host and avoid extinction. However, the definition of *T. gondii* virulence in laboratory inbred mice does not provide an explanation for virulent strains persistence in nature, since they all lead to lethal infections.

Two independent groups identified specific wild-derived *M. musculus musculus* and *M. musculus castaneus* strains which survive infection with virulent *T. gondii* strains and develop brain cysts (7, 62). Their resistance is correlated with specific alleles of the extremely polymorphic host Immunity-Related GTPase *Irgb2-b1*. Resistance-associated IRGb2-b1 has been shown to bind and inhibit the parasite main virulence factor ROP5 (7, 115). *Irg* sequences in laboratory mice strains are highly conserved due to the extensive inbreeding process, which makes these models not suitable systems to mimic natural infection. On the contrary, the identified wild-derived *M. musculus* subspecies surviving infection with virulent *T. gondii* genotypes and carrying high *Irg* diversity can potentially act as reservoir and allow further transmission to cats.

However, *M. musculus* might not be the most relevant intermediate host for *T. gondii*. Several studies conducted in Europe showed that the diet of feral domestic and wild cats consist mostly of *M. glareolus*, *Microtus* spp. and *Apodemus* spp. rather than *Mus* spp. The same species have also a higher prevalence of *T. gondii* infection compared to the previously examined *Mus* spp. Furthermore, there is evidence that these non-murine rodents are less susceptible to virulent *T. gondii* strains which eventually form brain cysts. As already speculated by Afonso et al., dietary habits of cats have a direct impact on their infection with *T. gondii* and this warrants further investigation (118). Therefore, the main aim of this study was to evaluate the potential for *M. glareolus*, *Microtus* spp. and *Apodemus* spp. to act as intermediate hosts for virulent *T. gondii* genotypes by resistance mechanisms involving IRGb2-b1-like proteins.

Different approaches are possible to unravel the link between *Irgb2-b1*-like genotypes present in nature and the *T. gondii* virulence phenotype. One strategy relies on genotyping naturally infected rodents in the wild as well as their pathogens. Whereas this might represent the ideal approach, it also presents drawbacks. First, many confounders in nature influence the outcome of infection, as for example concomitant infections, age and immune status of the host. Knowing the impact of each of these variables for developing a reliable model requires a deep knowledge of the studied population, a highly prevalent pathogen and a large sample size. Examples are given by the correlation between Tnf-α and *Mx2* expression and infection with helminths/hantaviruses (119, 120), or cytokines' genetic diversity and infection with several pathogens (121), both studies performed in a extensively studied population of *M. agrestis* in UK. The outcome of these studies is the likelihood that a certain factor is either directly or indirectly involved in infection with the pathogen. In a second approach the natural variability is transferred in an *in vitro* setting, by cloning the gene of interest from different wild individuals in a homogeneous host system. This approach allows a reduction in the sample size needed and causes an observable effect of the introduced gene, and has been used previously, for example to study the species specificity of Canine Distemper Virus (122). Both approaches can also be combined to formally assess the impact of a putative target emerged from an explorative analysis. In the specific case of IRG-mediated host resistance, pathogen infection is not only influenced by sequence diversity but expression levels play an equally crucial role. For example resistance-associated *Irgb2-b1* alleles were also more expressed than susceptibility-associated ones (7). Further, polymorphisms in the promoter region of *Irgb10* result in higher expression levels in a mouse laboratory strain, and is directly related to resistance to *C. trachomatis* (123). Therefore, in order to evaluate the effect of solely *Irg* polymorphisms, we need to control their expression levels. Overall these considerations convinced us in adopting the second approach, with cloning of *Irgb2-b1*-like genes from several wild rodents into *Mus musculus* Flp-In-3T3 fibroblasts. Since the latter were generated from inbred mice we expected these cells to encode for the *T. gondii* susceptibility-associated *Irgb2-b1* genotype, consequently to allow virulent parasite proliferation. Cloning of a resistance-conferring *Irgb2-b1*-like gene should mediate rupture of the parasitophorous vacuole membrane and cause parasite death. Flp-In-3T3 cells also allow a site-specific integration of transfected genes which results in comparable expression levels. This established cell culture-based system will allow me to evaluate the infection phenotype associated with *Irgb2-b1*-like genes from wild rodents.

In Chapter 1 I assessed the diversity of *Irgb2-b1*-like genes in samples across Germany from wild rodents of *M. glareolus*, *Microtus* spp. and *Apodemus* spp. Similarly to Lilue et al. in their study on wild-derived *M. musculus*, I expected a high diversity between and within these rodent species sequences. Selected *Irgb2-b1*-like genes were stably transfected into Flp-In-3T3 fibroblasts, starting from the positive control *Irgb2-b1*$_{CIM}$ with the resistance-associated CIM allele and the negative control *Irgb2-b1*$_{Bl6}$ with the susceptible allele from inbred mice. The created cell lines were observed in the context of virulent and avirulent *T. gondii* infection.

In Chapter 2 I produced and characterized a recombinant vole IFN-γ (124). Working with non-model organisms poses special challenges as the lack of reliable genomic references and reagents, like the crucial cytokine IFN-γ. Because of our interest in IFN-γ-induced genes and the availability of vole-derived cell systems, access to this cytokine was a prerequisite for the project. Due to the phylogenetic distance between voles and *Muridae* indicated in Fig. 2, we expected and initially proved lack of cross-reactivity of the murine IFN-γ on vole-derived cells. Thus, the vole cytokine was produced by recombinant expression in *E. coli* and its activity validated by several means.

In Chapter 3 I studied the IFN-γ-mediated resistance of different *M. glareolus*-derived systems to infection with virulent and avirulent *T. gondii* strains. Given *M. glareolus* less susceptibility to virulent parasite infection from *in vivo* studies compared to *Mus* spp., we expected vole cells to display a resistant phenotype. Similarly, resistant phenotype was expected against avirulent strains which do not cause acute toxoplasmosis in these rodent species. For this purpose, I established novel hematopoietic and non-hematopoietic cell cultures from *M. glareolus*, like Bone Marrow-Derived Macrophages and primary fibroblasts cultures, which are frequently used cell types in *T. gondii* research.

Taken together these results contribute to assess the ecological potential of rodent species as *M. glareolus*, *Microtus* spp. and *Apodemus* spp. as intermediate hosts for virulent *T. gondii* in Europe and their subsequent transmission to cats.

4. Materials

4.1 Media and agar

Tab. 3. Media and agar

Name	Composition
DMEM cell culture medium	DMEM *high glucose* (4.5 g/l) with sodium pyruvate and stable glutamine added with 1 or 10 % heat-inactivated FCS and 100 µg/ml Pen/Strep (1x)
Cell freezing medium	90 % (v/v) of either complete DMEM cell culture medium or FCS added with 10 % DMSO
Hogness freezing medium (10x)	36 mM K_2HPO_4; 13 mM KH_2PO_4; 20 mM Na-citrate; 10 mM $MgSO_4$; 40 % (v/v) glycerol (pH 7.5)
LB medium	10 g/l Bacto Tryptone; 5 g/l yeast extract; 10 g/l NaCl (pH 7.0)
2xYT medium	16 g/l Bacto Tryptone; 10 g/l yeast extract; 5 g/l NaCl (pH 7.0)
SOB medium	20 g/l Bacto Tryptone; 5 g/l yeast extract; 0.5 g/l NaCl; 2.5 mM KCl; 10 mM $MgCl_2$ (pH 7.0)
SOC medium	SOB-medium added with 20 mM glucose
DMEM medium for LDH assay	DMEM *high glucose* (4.5 g/l) and stable L-glutamine without sodium pyruvate and phenol red added with 1 % of heat-inactivated FCS and 100 µg/ml Pen/Strep (1x)

4.2 Buffers and solutions

Tab. 4. Buffers and solutions

Name	Composition
Inoue transformation buffer	55 mM $MnCl_2*4H_2O$; 15 mM $CaCl_2 \cdot 2H_2O$; 250 mM KCl; 10 mM PIPES (pH 6.7)
Crystal violet dye solution	0.2 % (w/v) in 2 % (v/v) ethanol
PBS	13.7 mM NaCl; 8.0 mM Na_2HPO_4; 2.7 mM KCl; 1.5 mM KH_2PO_4 (pH 7.4)
TBS	150mM Tris; 20mM NaCl (pH 7.6)
TAE electrophoresis buffer	40 mM Tris; 20 mM acetic acid; 1 mM EDTA
Permeabilization buffer	100 mM glycine und 0.25 % (v/v) Triton X-100 in PBS (pH 7.2)
Fixing solution	4 % (v/v) formaldehyde; 250 mM NaCl in PBS
Phosphoprotein lysis solution	10 mM Tris, 150 mM NaCl, 1 % TX-100, 1 % Na-DOC (pH 7.2)
Laemmli solution	250 mM Tris, 25 % (v/v) glycerol. 7.5 % (w/v) SDS, 0.25 mg/ml bromphenol blue, 12.5 % (v/v) ß-mercaptoethanol in ddH2O

Intracellular (IC) buffer (10x)	5 mM NaCl; 142 mM KCl; 2mM EGTA; 1 mM MgCl2; 5.6 mM glucose; 25 mM HEPES-KOH (pH 7.2)
Direct Blue 71 (DB71) whole protein staining	8 % (v/v) of 0.1 % DB71 stock solution in 40 % ethanol / 10% acetic acid solution
DB71 destaining solution	50 % (v/v) absolute ethanol, 15 % (v/v) 1M NaHCO$_3$, in ddH$_2$O
Bacteria lysis buffer	25 mM Tris; 500 mM NaCl; 10 mM imidazole (pH 7.5)
Lysis buffer for luciferase assay (5x)	125 mM H$_3$PO$_4$, 10 mM DTT, 10 mM CDTA, 50 % glycerol, 5 % TX-100, in ddH$_2$O (pH 7.8)
Luciferase assay reagent stock solution	20 mM Tricine, 1.07 mM (MgCO$_3$)$_4$Mg(OH)$_2$*5H20, 2.67 mM MgSO$_4$*7 H$_2$O, 0.1 mM EDTA, in ddH$_2$O (pH 7.8)

Tab. 5. Antibiotics and their used concentration

All antibiotics were diluted in ddH$_2$O.

Antibiotic	Stock concentration [mg/ml]	Working concentration [µg/ml]
Doxycycline	200	0.2
Timentin	50	25
Kanamycin	50	50
Blasticidin	10	20
Hygromycin B	50	200
Amphotericin B	25	0.25

4.3 Enzymes, proteins and antibodies

4.3.1 Enzymes and proteins

All enzymes used in this work (*Q5® High-Fidelity DNA Polymerase*, restriction enzymes, T4 DNA ligase, Antarctic Phosphatase) were bought from New England Biolabs GmbH (Frankfurt am Main, D). Exception were: the Dream*Taq* DNA polymerase and Exonuclease I (Thermo Fisher Scientific Inc., Karlsruhe, D); Shrimp Alkaline Phosphatase (SAP) from (Amersham, Freiburg, D);

The recombinant mouse IFN-γ was reconstituted in 1 ml sterile ddH$_2$O supplemented with 0.1 % bovine serum albumin (BSA) and stored in aliquots at -20°C (100 U = 20 ng).

The produced rec*Mg*IFN-γ protein solution was supplemented with 0.1% BSA and antibiotics (P/S) and stored in aliquots at -80°C.

4.3.2 Antibodies

Tab. 6. Antibodies and their used concentrations. WB: Western Blot; IF: Immunofluorescence assay; Cyt: Flow cytometry.

Antibody (origin)	Manufacturer	Dilution
anti-phopshoTyr701-STAT1 (rabbit mAb)	Cell Signaling Technology Inc., MA,USA	WB 1:1,000 IF 1:50
anti-phopshoSer727-STAT1 (mouse pAb)	Cell Signaling Technology Inc., MA,USA	IF 1:100
anti-STAT1 (rabbit pAb)	Cell Signaling Technology Inc., MA,USA	WB 1:1,000
anti-ß-actin (rabbit)	Cell Signaling Technology Inc., MA,USA	WB 1:3,000
anti-6His-tag (mouse mAb)	Linaris GmbH, Dossenheim, D	WB 1:2,000
anti-HA-tag (rat)	Roche Diagnostics GmbH, Berlin, D	IF 1:400 WB 1:500
anti-rabbit IgG (H+L) PO (goat)	Jackson ImmunoResearch Europe Ltd., UK	WB 1:3,000
anti-mouse IgG (H+L) PO (goat)	Dianova GmbH, Hamburg, D	WB 1: 2,000
anti-rat IgG (H+L) PO (donkey)	Jackson ImmunoResearch Europe Ltd., UK	WB 1:4,000
anti-rabbit Alexa Fluor® 488 (goat)	Thermo Fisher Scientific Inc., Karlsruhe, D	IF 1:1,000
anti-rat Cy5 (goat)	Dianova GmbH, Hamburg, D	IF/Cyt 1:500
anti-SAG1 (llama serum)	Preclinics Postdam	IF 1:500
anti-llama IgG Dylight 594 (goat)	Antibodies-online GmbH, Aachen, D	IF 1:300
anti-IRGB1 954/3 (rabbit serum)	Jonathan Howard, Instituto Gulbenkian de Ciência, Oeiras, P	IF 1:4,000
anti-IRGa6 165/3 (rabbit serum)	Jonathan Howard, Instituto Gulbenkian de Ciência, Oeiras, P	IF 1:8,000
anti-IRGb6 141/3 (rabbit serum)	Jonathan Howard, Instituto Gulbenkian de Ciência, Oeiras, P	IF 1:4,000
anti-IRGb6 TGTP A-20 (goat pAb)	Santa Cruz Biotechnology Inc., TX, USA	IF 1:50
anti-GRA7 (rabbit)	David Sibley, Washington University St. Louis, WA, USA	IF 1:1,000
anti-CD68/SR-D1 (mouse)	Novus Biologicals, Centennial, CO, USA	Cyt 1:10
anti-F4/80 (rat)	Santa Cruz Biotechnology Inc., TX, USA	Cyt 1:50
anti-mouse IgG PE (donkey)	Dianova GmbH, Hamburg, D	Cyt 1:100

4.4 Plasmids and oligonucleotides

4.4.1 Plasmids

Tab. 7. Plasmids

Plasmid (length)	Source and characteristics	AB-resistance
pASG-IBA33 (3,181 bp)	IBA Göttingen, Germany. Used for cloning of MgIFN-γ.	Amp
pQE90S-LEA (4,426 bp)	GenExpress GmbH (Berlin, Germany). Contains the TGME49_076870 *T. gondii* sequence in frame with a C-terminal 6His-tag used for production of LEA870 negative control.	Amp
pcDNA™ 6/TR (6,662 bp)	Invitrogen™ Corporation, Carlsbad, CA, USA. Used for cloning of BsdR gene in pGAS-Luc plasmid.	Bsd
pGAS-Luc (5,744 bp)	Stratagene. It expresses the firefly luciferase gene under the control of a promoter encoding a human γ-interferon-Activation Sites (GAS).	Amp
pGW1H-bl6-IrgB2B1-Flag (7,653 bp)	Jonathan Howard, Instituto Gulbenkian de Ciência, Oeiras, P. Used to clone the *Irgb2-b1*$_{BL6}$ gene into pFS-1 vector.	Amp
pGW1H-bl6-IrgB2B1-Flag-CIM (7,653 bp)	Jonathan Howard, Instituto Gulbenkian de Ciência, Oeiras, P. Used to clone the *Irgb2-b1*$_{CIM}$ gene into pFS-1 vector.	Amp
pUC19 (2,686 bp)	Standard cloning vector with *multiple cloning site*, LacZα.	Amp
pmaxGFP® (3,486 bp)	Lonza GmbH, Basel (CH). Expression of a GFP protein under the CMV promoter. Used as control for transfection efficiency.	Kan
pOG44 (5,785 bp)	Flp recombinase expression vector designed for use with the Flp-In™ System. When cotransfected with the pcDNA5/FRT plasmid into a Flp-In mammalian host cell line, like Flp-In™-3T3, the expressed Flp recombinase under a CMV promoter mediates integration of the pcDNA5/FRT vector containing the gene of interest into the genome via Flp Recombination Target (FRT) sites. Invitrogen™ Corporation, Carlsbad, CA, USA.	Amp

4.4.2 Oligonucleotides

Tab. 8. Oligonucleotides

Oligonucleotides	Sequence (5' -> 3')
Bsd Fw	TCATGATAATAATGGTTTCTTAGACCAGACATGATAAGATACATTG
Bsd Rev	ATTTCCCCGAAAAGTGCCACCTGACGAATGTGTGTCAGTTAGGG
B2-3' Fw	AAAGAAGAGCTTYTCACAG
B1-5' Rev	TCAGAGAGGATTTTRCTTTC
L-Ywhaz	GATGAAGCCATTGCTGAACTTGA
R-Ywhaz	GCCGGTTAATTTTCCCCTCCT
Cyt B Fw	TCATCMTGATGAAAYTTYGG
Cyt B Rev	ACTGGYTGDCCBCCRATTCA
Irgb2 Fw	ATGGGTCAGWCYTCCTCTTCTAC
Irgb2 Rev	CTGTGARAAGCTCTTCTTT
Irgb1 Fw	GAAAGYAAAATCCTCTCTGA
Irgb1 Rev	CATYSCTGYTTCCCAGTATTC
Irgb2 Slice Fw	TTTCTAGAGGCAAGGAAGCTCTTCGATGGGTCAGWCYTCCTCTTCTAC
Irgb2 Slice Rev	TTAAGCTTGCTTTCCTTGCTCTTCGTGTGARAAGTTCTTCTTT
b1f4 Slice Rev	TTAAGCTTGCTTTCCTTGCTCTTCGTCCCATYSCTGYTTCCCAGTATTC
b1f3 Slice Fw	TTTCTAGAGGCAAGGAAGCTCTTCGGAAAGYAAAATCCTCTCTGA
Irqb2qF1	CTGAACATTGCAGTGATGGG
Irqb2qR1	GGTCCCACAGTGTCACACT
Irqb1qF1	TCCATACCCACACCCAAAGC
Irqb1qR1	CAGGCAGGTCCCATATTGTCA
B2-3' Fw	AAAGAAGAGCTTYTCACAG
B1-5' Rev	TCAGAGAGGATTTTRCTTTC

4.5 Commercial kits

Tab. 9. Commercial kits

Name	Manufacturer
BigDye® Terminator v3.1 Cycle Sequencing Kit	Applied Biosystems, Carlsbad, CA, USA
DNA Clean & Concentrator™	Zymo Research Europe, Freiburg, D

Zyppy[TM] *Plasmid Miniprep Kit*	Zymo Research Europe
PureLink® HiPure Plasmid Midiprep Kit	Life Technologies GmbH, Darmstadt, D
Pierce[TM] *660nm Protein Assay Reagent*	ThermoFisher Scientific GmbH, Schwerte, D
PrimeScript[TM] *RT-PCR Kit*	Takara Bio Inc., Kusatsu, JAP
PrimeSTAR® GXL DNA Polymerase	Takara Bio Inc., Kusatsu, JAP
Maxima SYBR Green/ROX qPCR Master Kit (2x)	ThermoFisher Scientific GmbH, Schwerte, D
RNeasy Plus Mini Kit	Qiagen, Hilden, D
QIAshredder spin column	Qiagen, Hilden, D
DNeasy Blood & Tissue Kit	Qiagen, Hilden, D
NucleoSpin® Tissue DNA extraction Kit	Macherey-Nagel GmbH, Düren, D
Zero Blunt® TOPO® PCR cloning Kit	Invitrogen[TM] Corporation
Dual-Luciferase® Reporter Assay System	Promega GmbH, Madison, WI, USA
Amaxa® Cell Line Nucleofector Kit R	Lonza GmbH
Agilent RNA 6000 Pico Kit	Agilent Technologies Inc., Santa Clara, CA, USA
QuantiFluor® dsDNA Dye System and *QuantiFluor® RNA System*	Promega GmbH, Madison, WI, USA

4.6 Bacterial, eukaryotic and *Toxoplasma gondii* strains

4.6.1 Bacterial strains

Tab. 10. Bacterial strains

Bacterial strain	Genotype and source	AB-resistance
DB3.1	Contains ccdB-CAT as insert; released upon SapI-digest which was used for SLiCE cloning.	Kan, CAM
JM109(DE3)	Contains plasmid pKD46 (Coli Genetic Stock Center #64672). Used to prepare SLiCE extract. Grows at 30°C. Promega GmbH, Madison, WI, USA	Amp
OmniMAX 2T1R	Sensitive to ccdB toxin, used for positive selection of cloned genes via SLiCE and Golden Gate assembly. Invitrogen[TM] Corporation	Tet

4.6.2 Eukaryotic cell lines

Tab. 11. Eukaryotic cell lines

Eukaryotic cell lines (catalog number)	Species	Description and source
BJ-5ta (ATCC® CRL-4001™)	Homo sapiens	HFF cells for maintenance of *T. gondii* strains. Cells were immortalized after transfection with human telomerase reverse transcriptase (hTERT). From LGC Standards GmbH, Wesel, D
NIH/3T3 (ATCC® CRL-1658™)	*Mus musculus* (domestic mouse)	Mouse Swiss NIH embryonic cells. From LGC Standards GmbH.
Flp-In™-3T3 (R761-07)	*Mus musculus* (domestic mouse)	Cell line with FRT recombinase site for site-specific gene insertion. More details in chapter 6.1.5. From Invitrogen™ Corporation.
BVK168	*Myodes glareolus* (bank vole)	Derived from the kidney of a single animal. Description of BVK168 cell line establishment here (125). From Sandra Eßbauer, Institute of Microbiology, Munich, D.
FMN-R (CCLV-RIE 1102)	*Microtus arvalis* (common vole)	Derived from the kidneys of two common voles. Received from the Collection of Cell Lines in Veterinary Medicine (CCLV) of the Friedrich-Loeffler-Institut, Insel Riems, D.
AAL-R (CCLV-RIE 1297)	*Apodemus agrarius* (striped field mouse)	Derived from the lungs of a single animal. Received from the Collection of Cell Lines in Veterinary Medicine (CCLV) of the Friedrich-Loeffler-Institut.

4.6.3 Toxoplasma gondii strains

Tab. 12. *Toxoplasma gondii* strains

All parasite strains were cultered in DMEM cell culture medium added with 1 % FCS and p/s and frozen in freezing media with 90 % FCS and 10 % DMSO (v/v).

Toxoplasma gondii strain	Genotype and source
RhßGFPmt	Express a green fluorescence protein in the mitochondria and the β-galactosidase enzyme.
Pru tdTomato	From Jonathan Howard, Instituto Gulbenkian de Ciência, Oeiras, P.

PruΔku80Δhxgprt	LDH2 promoter-driven GFP. Pru-Δhxgprt-GFP was initially established (126) and ku80 subsequently deleted (127). From Martin Blume (Robert Koch-Institut).

4.7 Softwares and databanks

4.7.1 Softwares

Tab. 13. Softwares

Softwares	Manufacturer
AxioVision Rel. 4.8.	Carl Zeiss Microscopy GmbH, Göttingen, D
Geneious® *11.1.5*	Biomatters Ltd., Auckland, New Zealand
GraphPad Prism 7.4	GraphPad Software Inc., La Jolla, CA, USA
i-control 1.10	Tecan Group Ltd., Männedorf, Switzerland
ImageJ 1.51g	Wayne Rasband, National Institutes of Health, USA; used Macros: Count_Plaques_Toolbox_7 (written by Prof. Seeber)
PS Remote	Breeze Systems, Camberley, Surrey, UK
ZEN 2012 (blue and black)	Carl Zeiss Microscopy GmbH, Göttingen, D
CytExpert 2.1	Beckman Coulter Inc., Brea, CA, USA
7500 Software v2.3	Applied Biosystems Inc., Foster City, CA, USA

4.7.2 Databanks

Tab. 14. Databanks

Databanks	Manufacturer
Basic Local Alignment Search Tool (BLAST) (128)	http://blast.ncbi.nlm.nih.gov/Blast.cgi
E. coli genotypes	http://openwetware.org/wiki/E._coli_genotypes
National Center for Biotechnology Information (NCBI)	Literature research
Toxo DB: The *Toxoplasma* genome resource	http://www.toxodb.org/toxo/

5. Methods

5.1 Molecular Biology

5.1.1   Nucleic acid extraction from mammalian cells and wild rodent tissue samples

5.1.1.1 Wild rodent samples collection and genomic DNA isolation

Wild rodent samples from Germany were collected and kindly provided to us from Dr. Rainer Ulrich (Friedrich-Loeffler Institute, Insel Riems, Greifswald, D). Rodents were killed shortly after caught and the entire small intestine was cut from each rodent. Tissues were preserved in 15 mL falcon tubes filled with PBS, and stored at -70°C.

Two DNA extraction kits and several protocols for genomic DNA (gDNA) extraction were evaluated: the *NucleoSpin® Tissue DNA extraction Kit* and the *NucleoSpin® Soil DNA extraction Kit*. Each sample was thawed at RT, 25 mg tissue cut out with a sterile disposable scalpel and weighted, washed extensively with sterile PBS buffer, then gDNA isolation was performed according to manufacturer conditions with a pre-lysis step of 2 h at 56°C. gDNA was eluted in 30 µl sterile ddH$_2$0 and stored at -20°C until use. gDNA amount was assessed at the *Quantus™ Fluorometer* with the *QuantiFluor® dsDNA Dye System* according to manufacturer instruction and its quality in terms of 260/280 and 260/230 ratios with the NanoQuant Plate™ at the Tecan reader. A sample was considered of good quality when the 260/280 ratio was around 1.8 and the 260/230 ratio 2.0-2.2.

Murine tandem *Irg* sequences as reference were kindly provided by Jingtao Lilue (Wellcome Sanger Institute, Cambridge, UK).

5.1.1.2 Nucleic acid extraction from mammalian cells

gDNA

Cell pellets were resuspended in 200 µl PBS supplemented with 200 µg/ml Proteinase K and gDNA was extracted with the *DNeasy Blood & Tissue Kit* following the manufacturer's instruction. Samples were eluted in 200 µl ddH$_2$O, the gDNA amount assessed with the *QuantiFluor® dsDNA Dye System* and they were stored at -20°C until use.

RNA

Cell lines RNA for RT-qPCR was obtained with the *RNeasy Plus Mini Kit* from direct lysis in either 6 or 24 well plates. The cell layer was washed once with cold PBS, then covered with 350 µl of RLT Plus buffer added with 2-mercaptoethanol and the plate left for gentle shaking on a rocking plate for 5 min, then extraction was performed as protocol. Samples were eluted in 30 µl ddH$_2$O, the RNA amount was assessed with the *QuantiFluor® RNA System* and samples stored at -80°C until use.

RNAseq samples preparation and assembly

AAL-R, FMN-R and BVK168 cells were grown in two T75 culture flasks each and, when at 70-80 % confluency, treated with murine IFN-γ (200 U/ml) and rec*Mg*IFN-γ (200 ng/ml) respectively or left untreated as control. 24 h after treatment cells were detached from the flask with either trypsin (AAL-R) or *Accutase* (FMN-R and BVK168). Whole cell RNA was extracted with the *RNeasy Plus Mini Kit*. Each cell pellet was resuspended in 350 μl of RLT Plus buffer added with 2-mercaptoethanol as manufacturer's instruction and first homogenized with a pestel cleaned in a solution of 3 % H_2O_2 in ddH_2O, then passed through a *QIAshredder spin column* to increase the RNA yield. After, the flow through was passed through a gDNA removal column provided by the kit and the rest of the protocol was followed as instructions. RNA samples were eluted with 52 μl of RNAse-free water provided with the kit in individually packed RNAse and DNAse -free vessels and immediately stored at -80°C. A first assessment of RNA quantity and quality at the *NanoDrop*® ND-1000 spectrophotometer confirmed a yield of 50-100 μg per sample and optimal 260/280 and 260/230 ratios. Furthermore, quality was assessed by electrophoresis (Bioanalyzer with the *Agilent RNA Pico Kit*) to confirm integrity of extracted RNA. All samples presented the maximum Rna Integrity (RIN) value of 10 and clearly visible bands of 5.8S, 18S and 28S rRNA. Finally samples were shipped on dry ice to the Beijing Genomics Institute (BGI, Schenzen, China) for RNAseq. All surfaces prior RNA extraction and the Bioanalyzer before use were cleaned with the RNase*Zap*™ RNase Decontamination Solution.

RNAseq was performed for the 6 samples using Illumina-HiSeq2500/4000. 42.5 million reads were obtained on average per sample (minimum: 38 million; maximum: 56.5 million). RNAseq analysis is currently being performed by Alice Balard (Heitlinger group, Humboldt-Universität zu Berlin, Berlin). Erroneous k-mers were detected prior to the assembly using rcorrector (129) and read pairs for which one of the reads was deemed unfixable removed (https://github.com/harvardinformatics/TranscriptomeAssemblyTools/blob/master/FilterUncorrectable dPEfastq.py). Adapters and low quality bases were trimmed from fastq files using TrimGalore! (http://www.bioinformatics.babraham.ac.uk/projects/trim_galore) with a minimum read length threshold set as 36 bp. Transcriptomes were assembled de novo for each rodent species using Trinity version 2.6.6 (130). Quality of the assemblies was estimated using three methods. First, N50 (define as follow: at least half of all assembled bases are in transcript contigs of at least the N50 length value) was calculated was calculated for all samples. Then, bowtie2 version 2.3.0 (131) and samtools version 0.1.18 (132) were used to align the trimmed reads back to their corresponding transcriptome. Finally, transcriptomes completeness was quantified using BUSCO (Benchmarking Universal Single-Copy Orthologs) version 3.0.2 (133) with the mamalia_odb9 database. In a total of 4104 BUSCOs, the number of "complete"/"fragmented"/"missing" genes for our three transcriptomes were 74.9% / 5.6% / 19.5% for AAL transcriptome, 75.2% / 5.3% / 19.5% for BVK transcriptome, and 74.0% / 4.8% / 21.2% for FMN transcriptome. Moreover, transcriptomes for FMN-R cells (*Microtus arvalis*) and BVK168 cells

(*M. glareolus*) are currently analyzed by guided assembly on the available *Microtus ochrogaster* genome (genome ID 10848). This part of the analysis is still ongoing.

5.1.2   Reverse Transcriptase

Reverse transcription of mRNA to cDNA for use in PCR or RT-qPCR was performed with the *PrimeScript*™ *RT-PCR Kit* according to manufacturer's instruction. Up to 1 µg RNA was processed per reaction. A positive control provided with the kit and a negative control without template were included in each experiment.

5.1.3   PCR – Polymerase Chain Reaction

The PCR technique to amplify target genes has been extensively used for different purposes all throughout the project. Depending on the application, different Taq polymerases, PCR approaches or programs have been used. These are described in more detail below. In order to determine possible contaminations of the components used, each experiment always carried a control in which no DNA was present. The verification of a successful PCR was carried out by means of a gel electrophoretic separation or sequencing.

Analytical PCR

The analytical PCR was used to check for the presence of certain DNA segments in a DNA template. This may be the detection of an insertion into a plasmid after cloning or else the integration of gene segments into a genome. By default, the *DreamTaq*™ polymerase was used using a 50 µl PCR mix 1x *DreamTaq*™ buffer (10x), 0.2 mM each dNTP, 1.25 U *DreamTaq*™ polymerase, circa100 ng DNA and 0.2 µM of each oligonucleotide Fw and Rev contained in ddH2O. Unless otherwise described below, the following PCR program was used: 94°C 300 s; 35 × (94°C 30 s; Tm - 5°C 45 s; 72°C 90 s); 72°C 300 s; 4°C, where Tm is the annealing temperature of the primers.

When high sequence accuracy was crucial, e.g. for subsequent cloning of PCR fragments, the *Q5*® *Hot Start High-Fidelity* DNA polymerase with proofreading activity was used. 25 µl PCR mix were prepared with 1x *Q5*® buffer (5x), 0.2 mM each dNTP, 0.5 U *Q5*® polymerase, circa 100 ng DNA and 0.4 µM of each oligonucleotide Fw and Rev contained in ddH2O. The following PCR program was used: 98°C 30 s; 35× (98°C 10 s; Tm - 5°C 15 s; 72°C 30 s); 72°C 120 s; 4°C, where Tm is the annealing temperature of the primers.

For long amplicons (>8Kb) the *PrimeSTAR*® *GXL* DNA Polymerase was used. 50 µl PCR mix were prepared with 1x *PrimeSTAR*® *GXL* buffer (5x), 0.2 mM each dNTP, 1.25 U *PrimeSTAR*® *GXL* polymerase, circa 250 ng DNA and 0.2 µM of each oligonucleotide Fw and Rev contained in ddH2O. The following PCR program was used: 94°C 300 s; 35× (98°C 30 s; Tm - 5°C 30 s; 72°C 150 s); 72°C 300 s; 4°C, where Tm is the annealing temperature of the primers.

Colony PCR

The identification of successfully cloned recombinant plasmid DNA from the *E. coli* strains was carried out by means of a colony PCR based on the use of intact cells as DNA template. For this purpose, bacterial cell material of a colony was transferred with a sterile 200 µl pipette tip into a PCR reaction vessel with 50 µl PCR reaction (see above "Analytical PCR") and suspended by pipetting up and down. Subsequently the same tip was used to smear the colony in a new LB agar plate with the required AB selection.

5.1.4 RT-qPCR – Reverse Transcriptase quantitative PCR

The relative amount of mRNA abundance of *Irgb2-b1* compared to the reference gene tyrosine 3-monooxygenase/tryptophan 5-monooxygenase activation protein zeta gene (*YWhaz*) was performed via RT-qPCR. Cells were seeded into 24-well or 6-well plates and when at 70 % confluency treated for 24 h with different dilutions of rec*Mg*IFN-γ, mouse IFN-γ, negative control rec*Tg*LEA protein or left untreated as control. Then medium was aspirated and cells were washed once with PBS, and total RNA was extracted and reverse transcribed to cDNA. PCR primers to amplify *Irgb2-b1*, B2-3'-Fw and B1-5'-Rev, were designed on available *Microtus ochrogaster* and *M. musculus* sequences. PCR primers to amplify the reference gene *Ywhaz*, L-Ywhaz and R-Ywhaz, were based on the homologous *M. agrestis* sequence reported previously (134). The amplicon extends over intron 4 with 1764 bp in *M. ochrogaster*, whereas the mRNA-derived product is 155 bp. These primers also bind to the respective *M. musculus* sequence. Real-Time PCR was performed with the *Maxima SYBR Green/ROX qPCR Master Kit (2x)* on an *Applied Biosystem ABI 7500 Real-Time PCR system*. All reactions were run in duplicate with a no-template control to check for contaminations. Each tube contained 1 µl of cDNA template (equivalent to 5 ng), 12.5 µl SYBR Green mix solution, 0.75 µl primer (75 µM each) and 10 µl H_2O for a total reaction volume of 25 µl. The PCR conditions were 2 min at 50°C, 10 min at 95°C and 40 cycles of each 95° for 15 s and 60°C for 1 min. Melting curve analysis was performed from 60° to 95°C at 1 % ramp rate with each step lasting 30 s to confirm presence of a single product and absence of primer dimers.

5.1.5 Agarose gel electrophoresis

The products of PCR amplification were mixed with 1:10 *Midori Green Direct* DNA dye and applied to 1-3% agarose gel in 1x TAE buffer. The electrophoretic separation was then carried out after applying a voltage of 100 V in a horizontal gel chamber until desired separation of the bands of interest was reached. Separation of the DNA bands was visualized using a UV transilluminator. *Midori Green Direct* interacts with the DNA and can be detected by its absorption at ~500 nm as a green fluorescent nucleic acid dye. The size of the bands obtained was determined by comparison with the DNA size standard *GeneRuler*™ *1 kb Plus DNA Ladder*. If, after identification of a desired DNA fragment, the band is isolated by excision for downstream applications, it is called a preparative agarose gel. In that case the agarose gel was visualized at 470 nm using a blue light LED illuminator to avoid UV-induced DNA damage. To extract the DNA from the agarose gel, the *Zymoclean™ Gel DNA Recovery Kit* was used and then the concentration of DNA assessed at the *Quantus™ Fluorometer*.

5.1.6   Cloning

There are a variety of methods available to generate plasmids. In addition to the classical cloning variant, the ligating of DNA fragments after restriction enzyme digestion, two further methods were used in this work: <u>S</u>eamless <u>L</u>igation <u>C</u>loning <u>E</u>xtract (SLiCE) and Golden Gate cloning methods. SLiCE is based on cloning via homologous recombination and the second relies on type II restriction enzymes. They are described in more detail below. The plasmid maps of selected plasmids are reported in the book.

Seamless Ligation Cloning Extract (SLiCE) cloning method

SLiCE cloning methods allows cloning in a single step reaction without need ad additional ligation step. It relies on the amplification of a gene of interest (GOI) with primers encoding for recombinase sites in overhangs. The same recombinase sites are present in the recipient vector. When the vector, the recombinase and the amplified gene are incubated together, the gene gets easily inserted in the vector. A complete description of the method is reported here (135). Buffer and extract were prepared following published protocol, aliquoted and stored at -80°C until use. This cloning method was used thoroughly along the project for cloning of *Irg*-like genes from wild rodents into the pES51-bl vector, but also to create the pGAS-Luc-Bsd plasmid for the establishment of BVK-LucA reporter cell line. Before cloning, the vector was digested for linearization for 1 h at 37°C, followed by 20 min 65°C restriction enzyme inactivation step. Dephosphorylation was performed with the Antarctic Phosphatase following the manufacturer's instructions. I used an insert:vector molar ratio of 6:1 for 1.2 Kb inserts (as single *Irg* exons and BsdR), 2:1 for 2.5 Kb long inserts (as tandem *Irg*) and 1:1 for longer inserts. Each tube contained the calculated amount of insert, 1.5 µl of vector (equivalent to 100 ng), 1 µl of SLiCE extract, 1 µl SLiCE buffer for a total reaction volume of 10 µl. The vessel was incubated for 1 h at 37°C, then transformed in OmniMAX 2T1R bacteria. Omnimax cells allow positive selection via CcdB (136).

Golden Gate assembly

The Golden Gate Assembly method is based on Type IIS endonucleases which cut out of the recognized sequence and leave sticky overhangs (137). This renders the method particularly useful for cloning purposes. This cloning method was used to clone *Irg*-like genes from the plasmid pES51-bl to pFS-1. We use restriction with the SapI enzyme which recognizes the GCTCTTC1/4 site. This RE site was introduced at the extremities of Irg-like genes via during the cloning in pES51-bl. I used an insert:vector molar ratio of 1:1. Each tube contained the calculated amount of insert cloned into pES51-bl vector, 0.38 µl of uncut pFS-1vector (equivalent to 89 ng), 1.5 µl Cutsmart buffer, 1 µl SapI enzyme, 0.75 µl ATP 20 mM, 1 µl T4 Ligase HC for a total reaction volume of 15 µl. The vessel was incubated for 1 h at 37°C, then transformed in OmniMAX 2T1R bacteria and selected via CcdB as previously explained. I observed that incubation at 25 °C, suboptimal temperature for digestion, allowed me to obtain more full-length tandem *Irg*-like genes. As explained in section 6.1.5.4, these genes contained SapI RE sites and a suboptimal digestion increased the chances to clone the full sequence.

5.1.7 Sequencing

Generated plasmid DNA or PCR products were checked for correctness by sequencing. First a purification step using either the *DNA Clean & Concentrator*™ *kit* or a 2:1 mix of *Exonuclease I* and *Shrimp Alkaline Phosphatase (SAP)* used according to manufacturer's instruction was performed. Sequencing with the *BigDye*™ *Terminator 3.1 Cycle Sequencing Kit* was used, which is based on the Sanger method. After carrying out a PCR reaction of the DNA to be sequenced with in each case one oligonucleotide, the sequencing was carried out in the in-house facility. A 10 µl sequencing reaction contained 1x ABI buffer (5x), 1 µl *BigDye 3.1*, DNA and 0.5 mM of the oligonucleotide in ddH2O. The DNA amount varied according to the template length following the facility's guidelines, i.e. 10-20 ng for 500-1000 bp long PCR products, 150-300 ng for plasmids. The following PCR program was used: 96°C 120 s; 25× (96°C 10 s; Tm -5°C 240 s); 4°C, where Tm is the annealing temperature of the primers. The oligonucleotides used for sequencing the respective plasmids are listed in Tab. 8. The sequencing results were evaluated using the program *Geneious*® *11.1.5*.

5.2 Microbiology

5.2.1 Culturing and freezing *E. coli* strains

The cultivation of the different *E. coli* strains was mostly carried out at 37°C (exceptions are reported in Tab. 10) and 250 rpm in LB medium (liquid culture) or on LB agar plates with addition of the corresponding antibiotics in the reported concentrations (see Tab. 5). For the permanent storage of the strains, 900 µl of an o/n liquid culture were mixed with 100 µl Hogness freezing medium and stored at -80°C.

5.2.2 Production of chemocompetent cells and heat shock transformation

For the amplification of generated plasmids or for the reintroduction of already existing plasmid DNA in bacteria, a transformation was carried out. For bacteria to be able to take up external (plasmid) DNA, they must be brought into a state of competence, which can be obtained by different means. All throughout this project chemically competent *E. coli* strains were created and heat shock transformation performed, allowing the DNA to pass through the heat shock created membrane pores and thus enter the cell.

According to the protocol of Inoue et al. (138), a colony of either OmniMAX2T1 or DB3.1 *E. coli* strain was transferred to a 25 ml SOB or LB liquid culture with appropriate antibiotic and incubated at 37°C and 250 rpm for 6-8 h in a shaking incubator. Three 1 L flasks filled with 250 ml each of LB medium (+ AB) were inoculated with 2, 4 or 10 ml of this culture. The subsequent o/n incubation at 18°C, also in a shaking incubator, ended after one of the three cultures assayed reached an OD 600 of 0.55. The respective culture was chilled on ice for 10 min before centrifuging the cells at 4°C for 10 min at 2500 *g*. The supernatant was discarded and the cells gently resuspended in 40 ml of ice-cold Inoue transformation buffer, which was then centrifuged as before. The buffer was removed and the resulting pellet was resuspended again in 10 ml of ice-cold Inoue transformation buffer, mixed with 750 µl of DMSO and, after mixing, incubated again on ice for 10 min. The suspension was rapidly pipetted in 100 µl aliquots into 2 ml reaction tubes and, after sealing, placed in liquid nitrogen. The prepared competent cells were directly stored at -70°C.

For the transformation an aliquot was thawed on ice, added with 10-50 ng of plasmid DNA or with the cloning reaction and cooled for 30 min on ice. Subsequently the heat shock of the mixture took place for 30 s at 42°C in a water bath. Cells were immediately cooled on ice then regenerated without selection by adding 500 µl SOC medium for 60 min in a rotary shaker at 37°C 250 rpm. For the selection of recombinant clones, each mixture was plated on LB agar plates (+ AB) and incubated at 37°C o/n. To identify the recombinant bacterial colonies after transformation, a colony PCR was performed. After transformation of plasmid DNA, the bacterial strain was frozen or the plasmid DNA was recovered. As a control, an aliquot of competent cells was always transformed with the same protocol without DNA to test the effect of the antibiotic solutions used. After the preparation of competent cells, the transformation efficiency was always determined. For this, 5 ng of pUC19 plasmid DNA were transformed, 1:10 dilutions of the transformed cell suspension were plated and the colonies counted in a suitable dilution. The transformation efficiency was determined according to the following formula:

$$Transformants\ per\ \mu gDNA = \frac{colonies \times totalV(\mu l)}{platedV(\mu l) \times dilutionfactor \times \mu gDNA}$$

5.3 Cell culture

5.3.1 Cultivation of eukaryotic host cell lines

Adherently growing cells were cultured in DMEM (1 % or 10 % FCS) under 5 % CO_2 at 37°C and subcultured when confluency was reached. For this purpose, the medium contained in the cell culture flasks (T75) was aspirated with a plastic straw and cells were washed twice with 10 ml of PBS. Cells were detached either by adding 1 ml of trypsin / EDTA solution (1x) or 500 µl *Accutase* detaching solution, followed by a ~5 min incubation at 37°C. After 10 ml of DMEM were added to the bottle, the cell suspension transferred to a 15 ml centrifuge tube and either transferred immediately in a new flask in case of *Accutase* or centrifuged for 4 min at 300 *g* for trypsin / EDTA. After discarding the supernatant, the cell pellet was resuspended with 5-10 ml DMEM (10 % FCS) by gently pipetting up and down. Depending on the desired application, the cell suspension was diluted in DMEM (10 % FCS) and distributed in T25 / 75 cell culture flasks or 6 / 12 / 24 / 48 / 96 -well plates. If a 24-well plate should be prepared for an Immunofluorescence assay (IFA), the plate wells were prepared with Ø 10 or 12 mm coverslips before adding the cell suspension. For all cell lines reported in Tab. 11 DMEM cell culture medium with GlutaMAX™ added with 10% FCS was used.

5.3.2 Establishment of *Mus musculus* and *M. glareolus* primary cell cultures

Bone Marrow Derived Macrophages (BMDM) and primary fibroblast cultures were derived from both *M. musculus* inbred laboratory mice and from a colony of outbred *M. glareolus,* the latter property of Prof. Dr. Umberto Agrimi (Istituto Superiore di Sanità, Rome, I) and kept at the in-house animal facility of the institute under the supervision of Dr. Michael Beekes. Mice were anesthetized in a chamber containing isoflurane and sacrificed by cervical dislocation. Rear legs, ears, tail, brain, blood and intestine collected for different purposes.

Monocytes were extracted from both femors according to established protocols in the lab. The *M. musculus* inbred strain C57BL/6 was used for BMDM extraction. The general monocytes yield was around $3*10^6$ per *M. glareolus*, at least 10 fold less compared to C57BL/6 monocytes, which might be due to the smaller dimension of vole bones compared to mice ones. Monocytes were put in Petri dishes and differentiated into BMDM for 5-7 d according to the established protocols (139, 140) with complete DMEM added with 15 % L929 conditioned media (containing the murine macrophage colony stimulating factor (mM-CSF), (141)) and additionally 20 ng/ml recombinant human M-CSF for *M. glareolus* cells, then frozen in 90 % FCS / 10 % DMSO until use. After thawing, complete DMEM with both growth factors was used for vole BMDMs and replaced with 1.5 % mM-CSF only during experiments, whereas murine BMDMs suffice the latter.

Primary fibroblasts were obtained from either ears or tail of the animals and processed following the protocol of Khan et al. (142). For this purpose the *M. musculus* inbred strain B6.Cg-Tg(Vil1-cre)997Gum/J (stock 008546, The Jackson Laboratory, Bar Harbor, ME, USA) was used. The optimal medium condition resulted DMEM added with 10 % FCS and P/S, and incubation at 3 % O_2 in the hypoxia chamber conferred a slight growth advantage over normal 5 % O_2 other than the resulting higher number of passages in cultures already reported in literature (143). Further freezing in freezing medium composed of 90 % FCS / 10 % DMSO granted higher viability than 90 % complete DMEM / 10 % DMSO.

5.3.3 Antiviral activity assay

The viral infection with VSV*ΔG(FLuc) and MHV68 whatever viruses were performed by Georg Kochs (University of Freiburg, Germany). *M. glareolus* BVK168 cells were seeded into 24-well plates and 6 h later treated with either recMgIFN-γ (1:200 and 1:1,000 dilutions, equivalent to 1 ng/ml and 0.2 ng/ml, respectively), with the control protein LEA (in concentration analogous to rec*Mg*IFN-γ) or left untreated for 16 h before infection. In addition, recombinant human IFN-αB/D known to be active on *M. glareolus* cell line was used as positive control (5 ng/ml) (144). Next, the medium was aspirated and cells were inoculated with 0.5 MOI of VSV*ΔG(FLuc), a VSV glycoprotein-pseudotyped, propagation-incompetent VSV replicon, expressing firefly luciferase (145). At 24 h post inoculation cells were lysed in 80 µl passive lysis buffer per well and luciferase activity determined in duplicates in a luminometer via the *Dual-Luciferase Reporter Assay System.*

5.3.4   Mammalian cells transfection

Transient transfection

Both reagent-based and physical transfection methods were used on different mammalian cell lines. All reagents listed in Table 15 were tested according to manufacturer's instruction and conditions optimized for each experiment.

Tab. 15. Tested transfection reagents

Reagent	Method	Manufacturer	Reference
25 KDa linear Polyethylenimine (PEI)	Cationic polymer-based	Polysciences Inc., Warrington, PA, USA	(146, 147)
PolyMag™ and *CombiMag*™	Magnetofection™	Chemicell GmbH, Berlin (D)	
TransIT-X2®, *TransIT-LT1*® and *TransIT-2020*®	Polymer-based	Mirus Bio LLC, Wisconsin (USA)	
jetPRIME®	Polymer-based	Polyplus transfection®, Illkirch (France)	(148)
Lipofectamine™ *3000*	Lipid-based	ThermoFisher Scientific	

Other than these reagents, also the physical transfection method electroporation was tested for Flp-In-3T3 cells. For this purpose, the *Amaxa*® *Cell Line Nucleofector Kit R* specifically suggested for NIH/3T3 cells was used. 10^6 cells and 5 µg of plasmid (corresponding to 0.78 pmol) were mixed in the supplied cuvettes in serum-free Opti-MEM™ medium, electroporated with the U-030 program in the *Amaxa*® *Nucleofector*® *II Device*, then plated after 10 min recovery time in 4 wells of a 24 well plate with complete DMEM. Not electroporated cells as well as electroporated cells without plasmid DNA served as controls.

Transfection efficiency was tested by means of transient transfection with the pmaxGFP® vector and with pFS-CIM both expressing green fluorescent proteins. 24 h post transfection all cells nuclei were stained for 20 min in the dark at RT with 1:500 Hoechst 33342 and 1:500 Propidium Iodide to stain dead cells, then cells were immediately analyzed at the fluorescent microscope. The transfection efficiency was estimated by the proportion of green cells on the total living cells and expressed as percentage. The transfection methods that resulted successful for pmaxGFP® transfection in Flp-In-3T3 cells were also used for transfected with pFS-CIM and cells were tested for expression of HA-tagged IRGb2-b1 via immunofluorescence assay.

Stable transfection

Since *Lipofectamine*™ *3000* was the only successful reagent for transient transfection of pFS-CIM, stable transfection was attempted only with this reagent. Protocol was optimized on manufacturer's instruction as follow. Flp-In-3T3 cells were seeded in a 24-well plate and when at 70 % confluency transfected with pFS-derived and pOG44 plasmids in a molar ratio 1:5. pFS-derived plasmid concentration was always 1 µg/ml (corresponding to around 0.16 pmol), 1.5 µl/well *Lipofectamine*™ *3000* was used and all reagents were diluted in transfection-optimized Opti-MEM™ medium. At least four wells of cells were transfected per condition and each experiment included a positive control with pmaxGFP® for successful transfection and a negative control without DNA. The following day cells were analyzed at the Observer fluorescence microscope for successfully transfected cells expressing a green fluorescent protein, then left growing further in the incubator. Two days after transfection medium was exchanged with fresh one supplemented with 200 µg/ml Hygromycin B to select for positive clones, and exchanged every three days (+AB) to remove dead cells and debris. Cells were expanded for two weeks under constant AB selection.

5.3.5 Maintenance of *T. gondii* tachyzoites

T. gondii tachyzoites were cultured with HFF cells (Human Foreskin Fibroblasts, BJ-5ta ATCC® CRL-4001™) as host cells in DMEM (1 % FCS) under 5 % CO_2 and at 37°C. Every second to third day ~ 0.5 ml of a freshly lysed tachyzoite suspension was transferred to a T25 cell culture flask with confluent HFF cells with a Pasteur pipette. In order to determine the *T. gondii* cell number, infected HFF cells just prior lysis were used. Cells were scraped off T25 or T75 cell culture flask, passed through a 25 G needle mounted on a syringe two to three times for lysis, then transferred into a 15 or 50 ml centrifuge tube and centrifuged at 100 g for 5 min. The supernatant was then transferred to a new centrifuge tube and again centrifuged at 300 g for 10 min. The supernatant was aspirated with a plastic pipette and the pellet resuspended in 500 µl DMEM (1 % FCS) and transferred in a 1.5 ml vessel. A serial 1:10 dilution in DMEM (1 % FCS) was prepared and parasites from a 10^2 or 10^3 dilution were counted using the C-chip counting chamber according to the manufacturer's instructions. For infection experiments appropriate amount of parasites were diluted in cell culture complete medium and applied of the cell monolayer, then 2 hpi medium was changed to remove parasites that did not invade host cells.

5.3.6 Immunofluorescence Assay

For immunofluorescence assays (IFA) 24-well plates were always prepared with coverslips (Ø 10 or 12 mm) and seeded with eukaryotic cells with or without *T. gondii* infection according to protocol. After the desired period, the medium was aspirated and the cell layer washed with 1 ml of PBS or TBS buffer (according to the Ab protocol) before the cells were fixed by adding 200 µl of 4 % PFA solution in PBS or TBS for 20 min at RT. After washing again with 1 ml of PBS, the cells were incubated with 200 µl of permeabilization buffer for 20 min at RT before adding 200 µl of 3 % BSA solution in PBS or TBS to the wells for 1 h at RT or o/n at 4°C. Then, using a curved cannula and forceps, coverslips were transferred upside down on parafilm on 50 µl of the appropriate first antibody dilution in 3 % BSA solution in PBS or TBS and incubated for 1 h at RT. Coverslips were then transferred back to the plate for three washing steps with 1 ml PBS or TBS 10 min each. Staining with the secondary antibody dilution in 3% BSA solution in PBS or TBS was performed similarly to the primary antibody for 1 h at RT in the dark. Again, coverslips were transferred back to the plate and 200 µl of a 1 ng/µl DAPI solution in PBS or TBS were pipetted into the wells for DNA staining and incubated at RT for 10 min. After three washing steps with 1 ml PBS or TBS 10 min each, coverslips were placed on slides on 7 µl *Fluoromount*™ and lightly pressed. After hardening, images were taken on the Zeiss Axio Imager Z1 / Apotome or at the confocal microscope Zeiss LSM780. Image editing was performed with the programs AxioVision Rel. 4.8. and ImageJ 1.51g. The antibodies used and the dilutions used can be found in Tab. 6.

For *T. gondii* intracellular parasite growth, parasites were stained with an-anti-SAG1 antibody and a minimum of 100 vacuoles per condition were counted.

5.3.7 Detection of IFN-γ-mediated cell death

Cytotoxicity assay

Necrosis is accompanied by lactate dehydrogenase (LDH) release whose detection is part of the cytotoxicity (or LDH) assay and is a proxy for necrotic cell death. NIH/3T3 and BVK168 cells were seeded in a 24-well plate, treated with the murine IFN-γ (200 U/ml) and rec*Mg*IFN-γ (200 ng/ml) respectively or left untreated as control. The day after cells were infected with a MOI 2 of syringe-lysed Pru tdTomato or RHβGFPmt parasites or left uninfected as control and DMEM medium for LDH assay was used to reduce interference with the measurement. 24 hpi the plate was gently spin down at 1,500 rpm for 5 min, 100 µl of supernatant transferred in a 96-well plate and the LDH amount quantified with either a commercial *Cytotoxicity Detection Kit* or homemade reagents according to the protocol of Ka-Ming et al. (149). A control well of medium only was inclueded to measure the background signal which was subtracted to all values. The assay sensitivity was assessed via titration of fully lysed cells with 1 % TX-100 treatment for 45 min as suggested by the *Pierce LDH Cytotoxicity Assay Kit* manual (Thermo Scientific). Samples were incubated 30 min RT in the dark, then absorbance at 490 nm with reference at 680 nm was measured at the Tecan reader. Each condition was done in triplicate per experiment. Values were normalized to the signal from fully lysed cells.

Sensitivity was assessed via titration of TX-100-killed cells, leading to a detectable signal with 5 % of cell death in both set-up (Fig 5). This result indicates that homemade reagents represent a cheap and equally sensitive alternative to the more expensive kit. Considering that the expected impact of murine cell death 24 hpi with avirulent *T. gondii* is around 25 % (7), we concluded that the assay was suitable to our purpose.

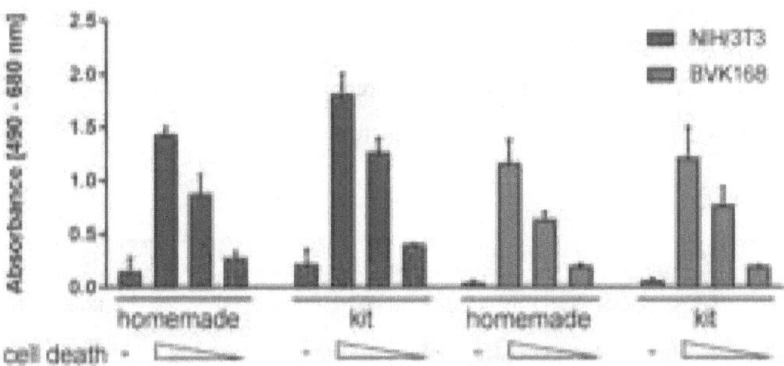

Fig. 5. Homemade and commercial LDH-detection protocols are comparable. NIH/3T3 and BVK168 cells were used to test the sensitivity of LDH detection comparing the protocol of Ka-Ming et al. (149) and the *Pierce LDH Cytotoxicity Assay Kit*. Cells were fully lysed with TX-100 and lysates were titrated to assess the sensitivity of the two protocols.

Propidium Iodide assay

Cells were either seeded in a 24-well plate or when available in a limited amount, i.e. *M. glareolus* primary fibroblasts and BMDM, in 96-well plate. After one day adaptation in culture, cells were treated with the respective murine IFN-γ (200 U/ml) –for Flp-In-3T3 and derived cell lines–, rec*Mg*IFN-γ (200 ng/ml) –for *M. glareolus* cell cultures– or left untreated as control. 24 h post treatment cells were infected with a MOI 2 of syringe lysed PruΔku80Δhxgprt or RHβGFPmt parasites filtered throught a 3 mm millipore filter to remove debris similarly to Niedelmann et al (150), or left uninfected. Medium was replaced with fresh one 2 h later to remove not invasive parasites. The proportion of dying cells 24 hpi was determined via a double staining with both a nuclear impermeable dye, Propidium Iodide (PI, final concentration 2 ng/ml), and a permeable one, Hoechst 33342 1:500 for 20 min RT in the dark. Images of around 500 cells per condition were taken at the Observer fluorescence microscope and the ratio PI⁺/Hoechst 33342⁺ assessed as proxy for cell death.

Cytometry-based assay

1x10⁶ *M. glareolus* BMDMs were seeded in 6-well plates and the day after treated with rec*Mg*IFN-γ (200 ng/ml) or left untreated as control. The following day cells were infected with a MOI 3 of syringe-lysed Pru tdTomato or RHβGFPmt parasites or left uninfected. Medium was replaced with fresh one 2 h later to remove not invasive parasites. 24 hpi the supernatant was transferred in a deep well 96-well plate and the cell layer washed with potassium (K⁺)-rich IC buffer (see Tab. 4) to avoid parasite premature egress due to osmotic stress (151). Cells were gently detached from the plate with 200 μl Accutase for 5 min 37°C and transferred in 96-well deep plates with the corresponding supernatant. Cells were spinned down at 500 *g* for 5 min and resuspended in 500 μl PBS added with 1 μl/well Violet LIVE/DEAD fixable dye (ThermoFisher Scientific GmbH, Schwerte, D) reconstituted on the moment and incubated for 30 min RT in the dark. Cells were spinned down at 500 *g* for 5 min and washed twice with 1 ml IC buffer, then fixed with 1 % PFA in IC buffer for 20 min RT. Cells were washed once and immediatly analyzed at the flow cytometer. A positive control of cells killed at 65°C for 5 min was always included, as well as a not stained well to remove background signal. 20,000 BMDMs were acquired, with gating performed on physical parameters.

5.4 Biochemistry

5.4.1 SDS-PAGE and immunoblotting

Cells were directly lysed in the plate for 30 min on ice with the lysis solution added with both proteases and phosphatases inhibitors. After centrifugation at the maximum speed for 5 min, soluble proteins were separated from the precipitate and collected in low binding vessels, and lysates quantified with the *Pierce™ 660nm Protein Assay Reagent*. Equal amount of protein samples were first added with loading Laemmli 5x solution added with inhibitors, then separated by standard SDS-PAGE and transferred to nitrocellulose by semidry blotting. A control for equal protein loading via the reversible Direct Blue 71 (DB71) staining according to the protocol of Hong et al. (152) was performed. After, non-specific binding sites were blocked for 1 hour with either 5 % dry milk or 3 % BSA in 0.1 % Tween-20 PBS solution. Membranes were incubated o/n at 4°C with the first antibody dilution in the blocking solution. After three washing steps with 0.1 % Tween-20 PBS solution, the membrane was incubated with horseradish peroxidase (HRP)-conjugated secondary antibody dilution in the blocking solution. Finally, after two washing steps with 0.1 % Tween-20 PBS solution and a single washing step with PBS, enhanced chemiluminescence reagent substrate of peroxidase was added and the signal detected using a luminescent image analyzer. The antibodies and dilutions used can be found in Tab. 6.

5.4.2 Luciferase assay

The BVK-LucA cell line was established as bank vole reporter for IFN-γ activity. For this purpose, BVK168 *M. glareolus* cells were transfected with PEI-transfection method (section 5.3.4 for details) with the plasmid pGAS-Luc-Bsd. The plasmid encodes for a firefly luciferase enzyme under the control of a promoter with GAS sites for STAT1 binding. The antibiotic Blasticidin was chosen for selection of transfected cells, thus the Blasticidin resistance gene (BsdR) encoding for Blasticidin-S deaminase was cloned from pcDNA6/TR into the final vector pGAS-Luc via SLiCE cloning. Transfected cells were selected with Blasticidin for two weeks before use.

For the luciferase assay BVK-LucA cells were seeded into a 48-well plate. After 24 h either serial dilutions of rec*Mg*IFN-γ or mouse IFN-γ and LEA or DMEM as controls were added and incubation was continued for 330 min or 18 h at 37°C as described previously REF. For infection experiment (Fig. 29) cells were infected with MOI 10 of RhßGFPmt or Pru tdTomato 3 h prior IFN-γ-treatment, or left untreated as control. The supernatant was removed, cells were washed once with PBS and 65 µl of lysis reagent was added to each well. The lysates were assayed using the *Dual-Luciferase Reporter Assay System*. 20 µl of the cell lysate was mixed with 100 µl of reconstituted luciferase assay reagent in a 96-well plate and the emitted light was measured in a Tristar LB 941 luminometer (Berthold).

For experiments in Fig. 29, a cost-effective and equally sensitive homemade luciferase assay reagent solution was used (already used in published work (153)). According to this protocol the luciferase assay reagent stock solution (Tab. 4) was added just before use with 33.3 mM DTT, 270 µM Coenzym A, 470 µM Luciferin and 530 µM ATP. The bioluminescence signal was detected as previously described.

5.5 Statystical analysis

Statistical analyses were performed using Prism 7 (GraphPad). Data were tested for normal distribution with the D'Agostino and Pearson normality test.

6.   Results

6.1   *Irgb2-b1*-like sequence diversity in wild rodents in Germany

In the first part of this project I explored *Irgb2-b1*-like genes' diversity in *M. glareolus*, *Microtus* spp. and *Apodemus* spp. across Germany. To this end I developed a cell culture-based system to study host cell phenotypes during *T. gondii* infection. The source of genomic DNA (gDNA) were intestinal tissue samples from wild rodents. Additionally, I had fortuitous access to different and rare wild rodents-derived immortalized cell lines established from rodents collected in Germany. In particular, I had two vole kidney cell lines, the *M. glareolus* BVK168 cell line (125) and the *M. arvalis* FMN-R cell line, as well as the striped field mouse *A. agrarius* lung AAL-R cell line. In addition, I used the commercially available NIH/3T3 embryonic fibroblasts cell line and, for stable cloning of *Irg* genes, the derived Flp-In-3T3 cell line, both derived from laboratory inbred *M. musculus*. All the mentioned cell lines are described in detail in Table 16.

Tab. 16. List of mammalian cells used in this part of the study.

Eukaryotic cell lines (catalog number)	Species	Cell type	Description and source
NIH/3T3 (ATCC® CRL-1658™)	*Mus musculus* (domestic mouse)	Embryonic fibroblasts	Derived from Swiss NIH mouse, LGC Standards GmbH.
Flp-In™-3T3 (R761-07)	*Mus musculus* (domestic mouse)	Embryonic fibroblasts	Derived from NIH/3T3 cell line. FRT recombinase site for site-specific gene insertion. More details in chapter 6.1.5. From Invitrogen™ Corporation.
BVK168	*Myodes glareolus* (bank vole)	Kidney epithelial cell line	Derived from the kidney of a single animal. Description of BVK168 cell line establishment here (125). From Sandra Eßbauer, Institute of Microbiology, Munich, D.

| FMN-R (CCLV-RIE 1102) | *Microtus arvalis* (common vole) | Kidney epithelial cell line | Derived from the kidneys of two common voles. Received from the Collection of Cell Lines in Veterinary Medicine (CCLV) of the Friedrich-Loeffler-Institut (FLI), Insel Riems, D. |
| AAL-R (CCLV-RIE 1297) | *Apodemus agrarius* (striped field mouse) | Lung epithelial cell line | Derived from the lungs of a single animal. From the Collection of Cell Lines in Veterinary Medicine (CCLV - FLI) |

6.1.1 Establishing the *M. ochrogaster* reference for *Irg*-like genes

One of the factors hampering research on non-model organisms is the lack of reliable genomic references (57). Despite continuous progresses, not much genomic and transcriptomic data are currently available and when available, they are not complete or badly annotated (58). If the situation is already complex for conserved genes, *Irg* genes which are among the most divergent ones in the mouse genome (154), pose further challenges. With the exception of *Irgc* on chromosome 7, *Irg* loci cover 3 240 Mb and 40 Mb long regions characterized by highly repetitive sequences that went through many duplication events and divergence cycles on murine chromosomes 11 and 18 (91). Characterization of this gene family was not trivial and, after a first pivotal work in 2005, its description is still ongoing (7, 91, 154).

To approach the complexity of *Irg* genes, we first analyzed the best available vole transcriptome, which is of *M. ochrogaster* (genome ID 10848), to identify the putative *Irg* loci and sequences and to design suitable primers for wild rodents' *Irg*-like genes amplification. When performing a Basic Local Alignment Search Tool (BLAST) of the *M. musculus* C57BL/6J (herein named BL6) *Irgb2-b1* sequence (*Irgb2-b1*$_{BL6}$, genome ID 52) against *M. ochrogaster* genome, we identified two *Irg*-like tandem genes (indicated by red arrow-heads in Fig. 6). The two tandems – named tandem 1 Irg (LOC101989451) and tandem 2 Irg (LOC101990019) – belong to two distinct loci and share higher similarity with the *Irgb5-b3* murine gene than with *Irgb2-b1*. The *Mus* spp *Irgb2-b1* tandems are encoded on chromosome 11. In *M. ochrogaster*, the *Irgb2-b1*-like tandems are encoded on chromosome 7. The conserved disposition of *Irg*-like genes in neighbouring loci and the presence of >6 kb long introns between single exons of the tandem make us confident in considering them putative *Irgb2-b1* genes (Fig. 6). Furthermore, the cDNA sequence, reported in full length in Fig. 9, has conserved residues typical of tandem *Irg* genes and important to develop their functions. The overall putative disposition of *Irg*-like genes in the *M. ochrogaster* genome on chromosomes 7 and 18 resembles the one on *Mus* spp.. Important genes involved in resistance to *T. gondii*, like *Irga6* and *Irgb6*, are also found similarly in this vole genome and transcriptome, as well as *Irg* genes with regulatory functions such as *Irgm*. BLAST of BL6 *Irg* genes against *M. ochrogaster* genome identified in total 21 putative *Irg*-like genes.

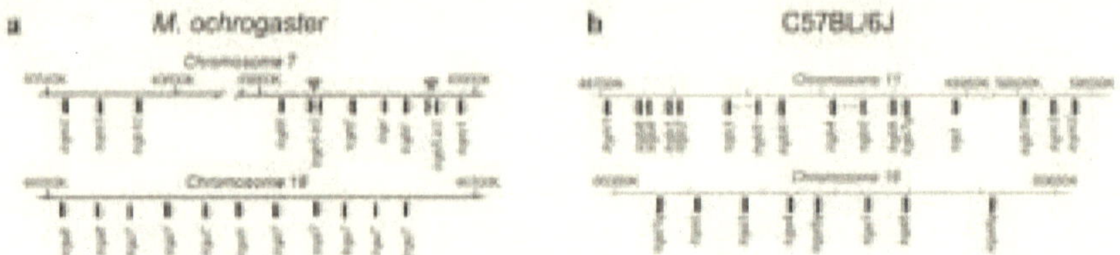

Fig. 6. ***Irg*** **genes are conserved in clusters in both** ***M. ochrogaster*** **and** ***Mus*** **spp. genomes. (a)** Schematic representation of putative *Irg*-like genes disposition on chromosomes 7 and 18 of *M. ochrogaster* (genome ID 10848). Red harrow-heads indicate the *Irg*-like tandem genes. **(b)** Disposition of *Irg* on chromosomes 11 and 18 of laboratory BL6 mouse genome. Figure from Lilue et al. (7).

Degenerated primers to amplify tandem *Irg*-like genes from wild rodents-derived samples were designed based on the consensus alignment between *Irgb2-b1*BL6 and the identified vole tandems as shown in Fig. 7. The *Irgb2* Fw primer ("Irgb2 Fw") starts with the start codon encoding for methionine, whereas the *Irgb1* Rev primer ("Irgb1 Rev") ends three amino acid (aa) upstream for reasons explained further in chapter 6.1.5.1. The big divergence around the splicing site in the middle of the sequence limited our possibilities for primer design. Thus, between the *Irgb2* Rev primer ("Irgb2 Rev") and the *Irgb1* Fw ("Irgb1 Fw") primer there are 117 bp which are not amplified by PCR of the single exons. The sequences are depicted in full length in Fig. 9 and primer sequences are reported in Tab. 8.

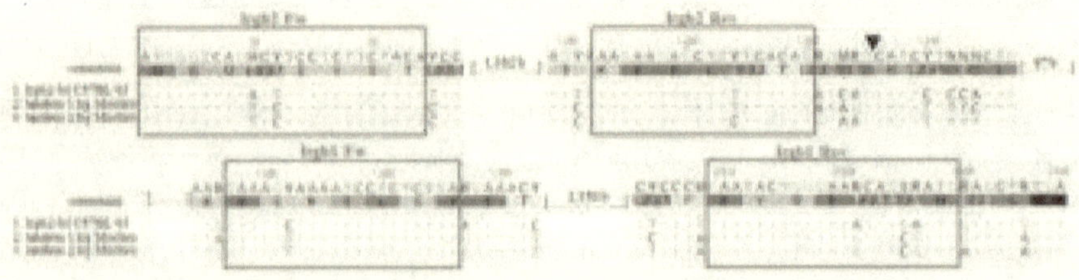

Fig. 7. Degenerated primers for ***Irg*-like genes amplification were designed based on** ***Mus musculus*** **and** ***M. ochrogaster*** **sequences.** The alignment between *M. musculus* BL6 *Irgb2-b1* and *M. ochrogaster* putative *Irg* tandem genes (genome ID 10848) was used to design primers. Red boxes highlight alignment and relative consensus used to design degenerated primers, with primer names reported above the boxes. Conserved residues are represented by dots and divergent ones are highlighted. The black arrow-head indicates the splicing site between *Irgb2* and *Irgb1*. Positions of the nucleotides relative to the alignment are indicated above the sequences.

6.1.2   *Irg*-like sequences from wild rodents-derived cell lines

Even though the best quality vole genome available is from *M. ochrogaster*, it is an American and not a European rodent species. Availability of the cell lines from Germany and of the recombinant vole IFN-γ (rec*Mg*IFN-γ, results in chapter 6.2 and Tab. 16 above), allowed us to obtain IFN-γ-induced tandem *Irgb2-b1*-like genes from German specimens of the considered *M. glareolus*, *Microtus* spp. and *Apodemus* spp.. The identified sequences can be used as better reference for tissue-derived sequences than *Mus* spp. and *M. ochrogaster*.

First, I amplified the whole genomic locus by PCR in all cell lines. Since both murine and vole references have tandem genes with different intronic sizes, resulting in ~9 kb and ~11 kb long gDNA, amplification of tandem *Irg*-like genes from wild rodents-derived cell lines was performed with the *PrimeSTAR® GXL DNA Polymerase* suitable for long amplicons. Two bands of the expected size were identified for inbred mouse-derived Flp-In-3T3 cell (lower and higher bands indicated by a black and red asterisk respectively on Fig. 8a). Similarly, FMN-R and AAL-R cells displayed two bands of analogous size, and BVK168 cells a single band of ~8 bb.

Following this, vole cells (FMN-R and BVK168) and murine cells (AAL-R and Flp-In-3T3) were treated for 24 h with 200 ng/ml rec*Mg*IFN-γ and with 200 U/ml mouse IFN-γ respectively, according to results presented in chapter 6.2 and as published (7, 91). Full length tandem *Irg*-like genes were PCR amplified with the same primer pair from mRNA reverse transcribed into cDNA. For all cell lines a 2.5 Kb long band was observed in treated cells but not in untreated controls (Fig. 8b, untreated controls not shown), confirming the IFN-γ induction of tandem *Irg*-like genes expression also in these species. These results confirmed the likely presence of similar *Irg* loci in *M. glareolus*, *M. arvalis* and *A. agrarius*.

Direct sequencing of the 2.5 kb PCR products revealed mixed bases in certain positions, indicating the presence of different products with the same size (example of FMN-R tandem *Irg*-like gene in Fig. 8c). These mixed nucleotides were observed for all tandem *Irg*-like sequences from wild rodents-derived cell lines, even for BVK168 cells which had a single band amplified from the gDNA, and sometimes resulted in amino acid differences (Fig. 8c). Mixed bases were observed from sequencing not only with primers designed on the amino (N-) and carboxy (C-) terminal, but also with primers designed within the sequences. These results indicate conservation of primer binding sites both within and at the exon extremities of *Irg*-like genes. To obtain single *Irg*-like sequences possible solutions were: 1) design of sequence-specific primers for each of these species' *Irg*-like gene 2) clone of the single amplified genes into a vector prior to sequencing. Given the lack of good quality genomic references for the rodent species in study, and considering that eventually the genes would have been cloned in mammalian cells, I opted for the second.

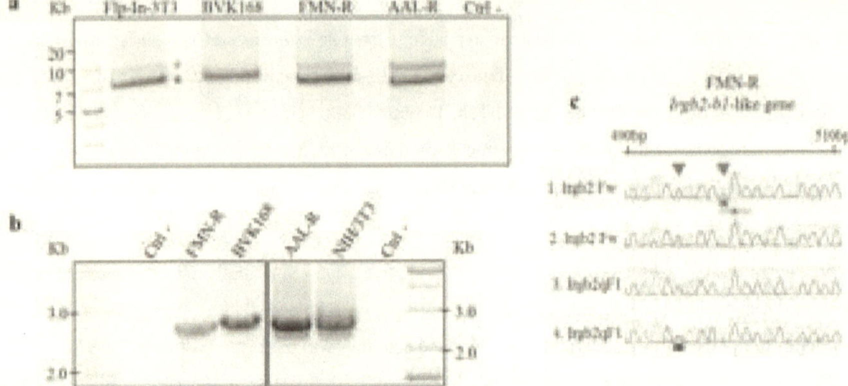

Fig. 8. *M. glareolus*, *Microtus arvalis* **and** *Apodemus agrarius* **have more than one tandem** *Irg*-**like gene. (a)** 0.5 % Agarose gel loaded with PCR amplified *Irg* and *Irg*-like tandem genes from gDNA of murine Flp-In-3T3, *M. glareolus* BVK168, *M. arvalis* FMN-R and *A. agrarius* AAL-R cells. Black and red asterisks indicate the smaller and larger band sizes respectively. **(b)** 1 % Agarose gel loaded with PCR amplified *Irg*-like tandem genes from cDNA of the same cell lines after 24 h IFN-γ stimulation. Untreated controls are not shown. Vole cells (BVK168 and FMN-R) were treated with 200 ng/ml rec*Mg*IFN-γ and murine cells (NIH/3T3 and AAL-R) with 200 U/ml mouse IFN-γ. First and last lanes with DNA marker (with sizes in kb given on the side). **(c)** Example of direct sequencing of *Irg*-like tandem genes' PCR products from FMN-R cells. Ambiguous bases are highlighted with red arrow-heads and indicate the presence of either heterozygotes or different genes with the same size amplified. The same PCR product was sequenced with two different primer pairs ("Irgb2 Fw" and "Irqb2qF1") twice as indicated on the left. Positions of nucleotides relative to the start codon are indicated above the sequences.

I cloned *Irgb2-b1*-like genes in the plasmid pES51-b1 prior sequencing. I adopted the convenient <u>S</u>eamless <u>L</u>igation <u>C</u>loning <u>E</u>xtract (SLiCE) method, which allows cloning of genes of interest in a single-step reaction. Requirement for the SLiCE cloning is amplification of the gene of interest with primers with overhangs encoding for recombination sites, to allow insertion of the gene in the vector via homologous recombination. Two tandems were successfully cloned from AAL-R cells, and a single one from BVK168 and FMN-R cells. However, sequencing data indicate the presence of more tandem *Irg*-like genes in the cell lines. Sequences of the cloned genes and alignment of these sequences are reported in Fig. 9.

Cloning was attempted also for the tandem *Irg*-like genes amplified from gDNA. However, cloning of these only yielded a few positive clones, i.e. from the band indicated with the black asterisk in Fig. 8a of Flp-In-3T3, FMN-R and AAL-R cell lines. The cloned FMN-R-derived sequence shared a higher similarity with *M. ochrogaster* tandem 1 Irg (LOC101989451) which also corresponds to the smaller genomic sequence. This and the cloned tandem from cDNA shared a deletion around 420 bp, which characterizes tandem 2 Irg (LOC101990019), although they diverge at many residues (not shown). The cloned AAL-R gDNA-derived sequence was identical to the cloned tandem 1 from cDNA (AAL-R tandem 1 in Fig. 9).

Cloned tandem *Irg*-like sequences from wild rodents-derived cell lines and published murine tandem *Irg* genes (*Irgb2-b1*$_{BL6}$, *Irgb2-b1*$_{CIM}$ and *Irgb2-b1*$_{PWD/EiJ}$) are reported in Fig. 9. The susceptible phenotype-associated *Irgb2-b1*$_{BL6}$ was used as reference in the alignment. All cloned sequences terminate with a methionine, two aa before the stop codon, for reasons explained in chapter 6.1.5.1. The *Irgb1*-like sequence of AAL-R tandem 2 gene is characterized by many stop codons, which may hint to the presence of a pseudogene. However, I cannot exclude that the presence of several adenine residues in a row (Fig. 37 in the appendix) induced a mistake in the polymerase activity and caused a frame-shift. Cloned *Irg*-like sequences have conserved GTPase motifs at the amino-terminal, like the α-phosphate-binding loop G(X$_4$)GKS and the DXXG motif (highlighted in red boxes in Fig. 9, (83)). The latter is not present in *Irgb2-b1*$_{BL6}$ and *Irgb2-b1*$_{CIM}$, and murine *Irgb2-b1* sequences also lack the nine aa-long insertion at the utmost amino-terminal. More deletions characterize vole sequences, like the one of four aa around the residue 830 as well as a smaller one of two aa right after the splicing site indicated with a black arrow-head in Fig. 9. All tandem sequences have a conserved histidine as first amino acid of the IRGb1 exon. I observed variability between these sequences, especially in the αD and H4 domains which interact with *T. gondii* virulence factor ROP5 in *Mus* spp., as well as in residues in position 245-318 and after the splicing site. In general, a higher diversity in the *Irgb2* exong compared to *Irgb1* was previously observed within murine genes and is through my work confirmed in other wild rodent species.

Fig. 9 (following page). High variability between murine and vole *Irg* tandem genes. Alignment of *Mus* spp. tandem Irg genes and tandem *Irg*-like genes cloned from wild rodents-derived cell lines. *Irgb2-b1*$_{BL6}$ was used as reference. Important domains and motifs are indicated in red boxes, and the splicing site by a black arrow-head. Conserved amino acids are represented by dots and divergent ones are highlighted. Amino acid positions relative to the alignment are indicated above the sequences.

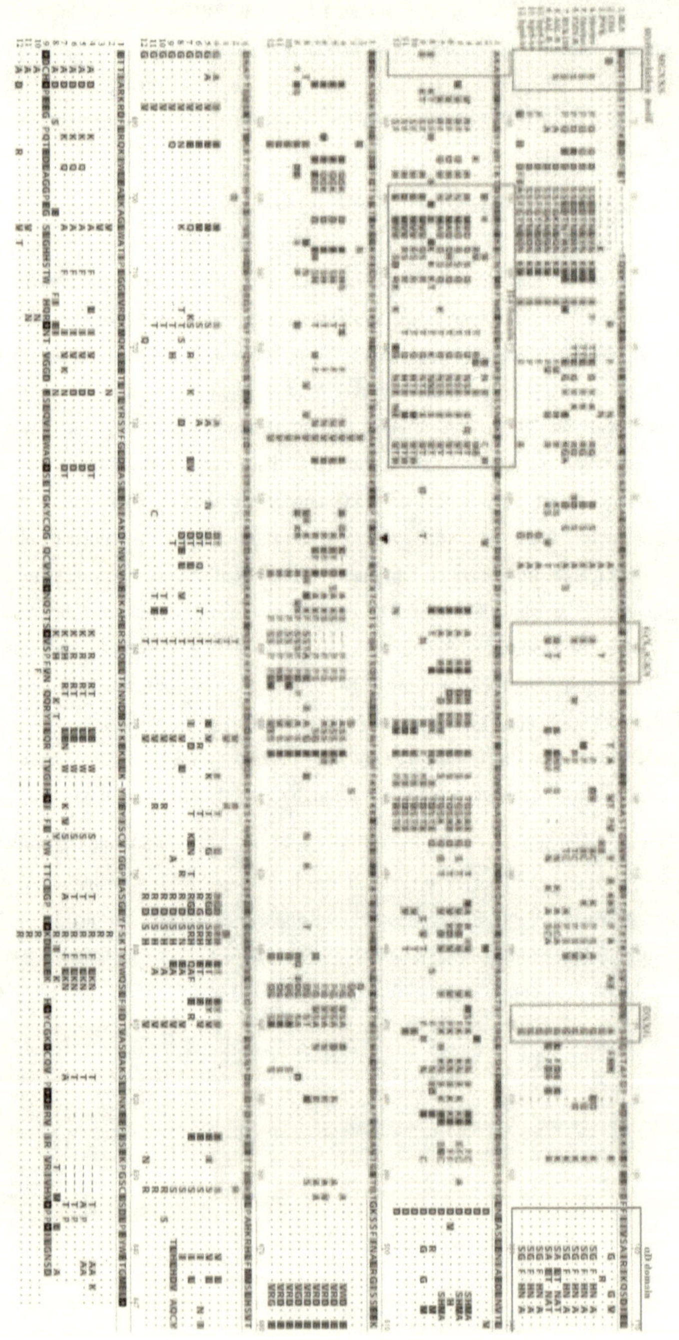

6.1.3   RNAseq data of *M. glareolus*, *Microtus arvalis* and *Apodemus agrarius* cell lines

Analysis based on binding of designed degenerated primer pairs skews the results towards sequences more similar to the reference sequence. In order to make an unbiased identification of *Irg*-like genes in the available wild rodents-derived cell lines, we performed an RNAseq analysis of the same, treated and not treated with IFN-γ. A complete list of prepared RNA samples is presented in Tab. 17. RNA samples with high yield (50-100 µg per sample) and good quality evaluated at the Bioanalyzer were obtained. Finally, samples were sent for RNAseq and results are currently being analyzed in collaboration with Alice Balard (Heitlinger group, Humboldt Universität, Berlin). Preliminary results of the *de novo* assembly explained in section 5.1.1.2 are reported. First, at least half of all assembled bases in each transcript are more than 2500 bases-long and more than 97 % of fragments were aligned as proper pairs in all three transcriptomes. Moreover, for each prepared sample more than 74 % of assemblies is recognized as full-length genes compared to a mammalia database (see section 5.1.1.2 for details), around 5 % as fragmented and 20 % missing. Overall, first indications point out to a good and uniform quality of the RNAseq data, which is a prerequisite for future transcriptomic analysis.

Tab. 17 List of samples prepared for RNAseq. Rec*Mg*IFN-γ was used in a concentration 200 ng/ml and mouse IFN-γ 200 U/ml; both treatments were performed for 24 h.

Sample #	Species	Cell line	Condition
1	*A. agrarius*	AAL-R	untreated control
2	*A. agrarius*	AAL-R	mouse IFN-γ
3	*M. glareolus*	BVK168	untreated control
4	*M. glareolus*	BVK168	rec*Mg*IFN-γ
5	*M. arvalis*	FMN-R	untreated control
6	*M. arvalis*	FMN-R	rec*Mg*IFN-γ

6.1.4   *Irg*-like sequences from wild rodents-derived tissue samples

6.1.4.1 Extraction of genomic DNA and rodent species determination

A subset of tissue samples from the collection available to us was selected for gDNA extraction. Two DNA extraction kits and several protocols for gDNA extraction were evaluated. The *NucleoSpin® Tissue DNA extraction Kit* allowed us to obtain high yield of gDNA with a less laborious protocol than the *NucleoSpin® Soil DNA extraction Kit*, therefore was the kit of choice for the processing of wild rodents tissue samples. gDNA yield and quality varied widely, supposedly due to contaminants in the intestinal tissue used. Many samples displayed almost undetectable gDNA amount and high impurity (in terms of 260/280 ratio measured at the NanoQuant Plate™). The part of samples considered suitable (260/280 ratio so-so) were stored for subsequent PCR reactions. First, the rodent species hypothesized by morphometric analysis at the moment of capture was confirmed by PCR amplification and sequencing of *CytB*, according to the protocol of Schlegel et al. (155). The latter is based on degenerated primers designed to amplify numerous small mammals' *CytB* sequences and allowed us to classify them at the species level. Initially PCR amplification lacked reproducibility, with the PCR products not always present despite applying the same DNA template and reaction protocol. The reason likely lies in the presence of phenol compounds in fecal materials, which potentially inhibits the reaction (156). The addition of Bovine Serum Albumin (BSA) greatly improved the PCR amplification yield (Fig. 10a) and was then applied to all PCR reactions with gDNA derived from tissue samples.

6.1.4.2 *Irg*-like sequences from wild rodents-derived tissue samples

I then proceeded to PCR-amplify and sequence *Irg*-like genes from the same tissue-derived gDNA used for *CytB* amplification. *Irgb2*-like and *Irgb1*-like genes were amplified with the degenerated primers designed based on both *Mus* spp. and *M. ochrogaster* genomes as described previously. Despite the addition of BSA and several steps of optimization of the protocol, only approximately half the samples generated a PCR product ~1.2 kb long (Fig. 10b). I thus cloned *Irgb2*-like and *Irgb1*-like genes in the plasmid pES51-bl via SLiCE cloning method previously explained. Amplification was most efficient for the primer pair designed to amplify the *Irgb1*-like gene and provided few *Irgb2*-like sequences. In an attempt to enlarge our repertoire of *Irgb2*-like sequences, I thus used the *Zero Blunt® TOPO® PCR cloning Kit*, which allows cloning of blunt end PCR products in a single-reaction step, to clone *Irgb2*-like sequences that were successfully amplified without SLiCE primers. These different cloning methods confirmed the presence of different alleles or genes amplified by the same primer pair, since the same PCR product produced up to four different sequences (e.g. 050_Aag in Fig. 11). However, the yield in terms of number of colonies was low with less than 20 colonies per amplicon. This is despite transformation of all the cloning reaction, plating of all the transformation solutions, and use of high transformation efficiency commercial bacteria). Considering the high cost of this approach, it cannot be considered optimal to explore *Irg*-like genes diversity. Amplification of the whole *Irgb2-b1*-like locus from gDNA was attempted, but was unsuccessful, likely due to poor DNA quality (data not shown).

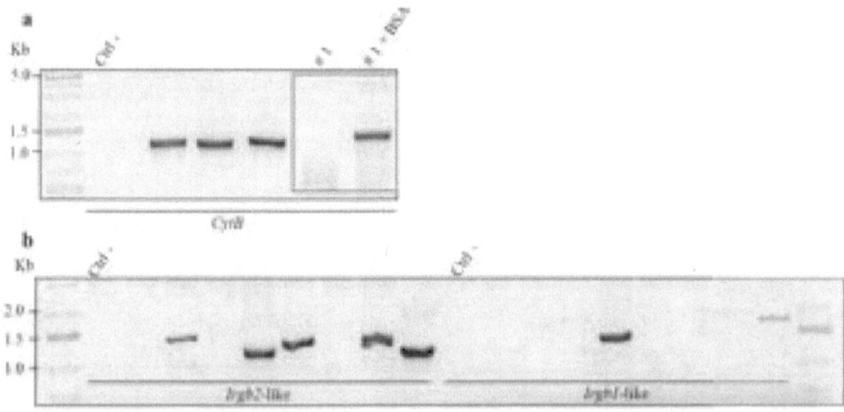

Fig. 10. The poor gDNA quality and diversity at the primers' binding sites might account for low PCR amplification yield. PCR amplification from wild rodents-derived gDNA of *CytB* and *Irg*-like genes. **(a)** 1 % Agarose gel loaded with PCR amplified *CytB* gene for rodent species determination. The red box highlights two lanes where the reaction was performed with the same gDNA template (sample #1) with and without addition of BSA 1μg/μl. **(b)** 1 % agarose gel of PCR-amplified *Irgb2*-like and *Irgb1*-like genes (with BSA). Midori Direct was used to visualize the ladder and the PCR products. First and last lanes are DNA markers (with sizes in kb given to the left).

Recently the group of Tobias Steinfeldt (University of Freiburg, Germany) showed that the IRGb2 subunit of IRGb2-b1 is responsible for mediating the resistant phenotype in *M. musculus castaneus* CIM cells and that the mechanism is based on binding of *T. gondii* virulent ROP5 protein (115). Therefore, it is reasonable to assume that resistance is accomplished by the 43 amino acids which are different between susceptible IRGb2$_{BL6}$ and resistant IRGb2$_{CIM}$. An alignment of 33 out of the 43 differential amino acids are displayed in Fig. 11 and compared to collected IRGb2-like sequences from wild rodents. We observed diversity between IRGb2$_{BL6}$ and approximately half of the residues in wild rodents-derived sequences. Some residues are conserved in all non-*Mus* spp. sequences, whereas others display a higher diversity, e.g. in positions 99, 151 and 180. Interestingly, the diverging residues in positions highlighted by red boxes are enriched at the putative interface with ROP5, as shown in the structural model of *M. ochrogaster* IRGb2-like binding to ROP5 (Fig. 12).

These results indicate that there is variability between and within rodent species' *Irg*-like genes, similarly to the differences in wild *Mus* spp.-derived sequences. Different residues are enriched at the putative interface with T. gondii virulence factor ROP5.

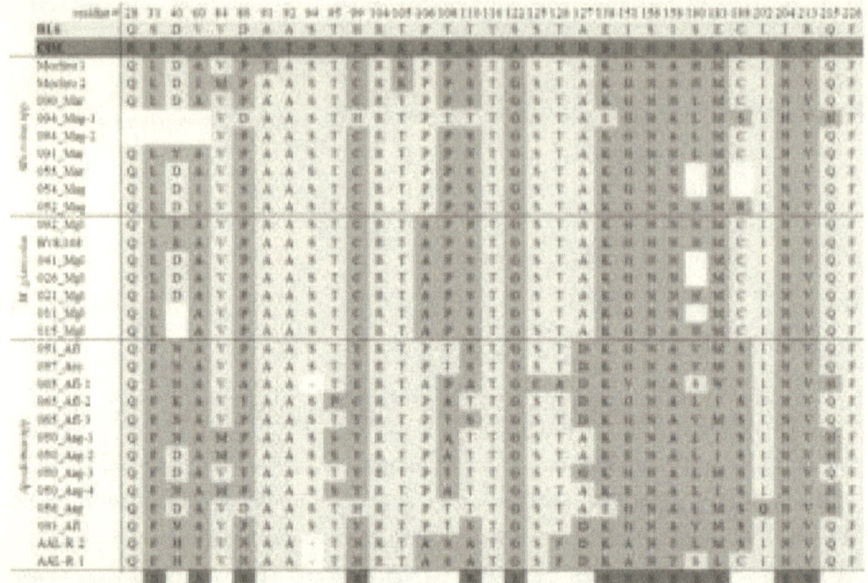

Fig. 11. Wild rodents-derived Irg-like proteins have high diversity in residues that vary between resistant and susceptible murine sequences. Amino acid alignment of IRGb2 and IRGb2-like proteins from susceptible inbred BL6, resistant *Mus musculus castaneus* CIM (CIM) and wild rodents of *M. glareolus*, *Microtus* spp. and *Apodemus* spp. Afl = *A. flavicollis*; Aag = *A. agrarius*; Asy = *A. sylvaticus*; Mgl = *M. glareolus*; Mag = *M. agrestis*; Mar = *M. arvalis*; Mochro = *M. ochrogaster*. Positions of the amino acid relative to murine references are indicated above the sequences. Residues conserved between the analyzed sequenced and BL6 are indicated in yellow boxes. Varying amino acids in the same position where CIM varies are highlighted in orange. The positions indicated by red boxes under the alignment refer to residues highlighted in the following Fig. 12. Missing residues due to inconsistent sequencing results are left blank and gaps are indicated by a hyphen.

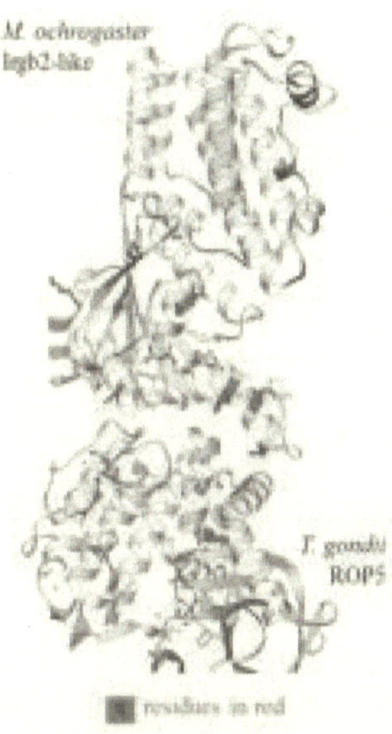

Fig. 12. Wild rodents-derived IRG-like proteins have high diversity in residues at the putative interface with ROP5. *M. ochrogaster* IRGb2-like residue (LOC101989451, genome ID 10848) was modeled onto mouse IRGa6 (PMID: 29788355) bound to Toxoplasma ROP5B (PDB: 4LV5). Residues in the positions highlighted in red in the alignment in Fig. 11 are indicated with the same color in the structure. The model was created using Swiss-Model (157) and the resulting model visualized with UCSF Chimera 1.1.3. (158). The structural model was created by Frank Seeber (Robert Koch-Institut).

6.1.5 Establishment of an *in vitro* system to study wild-derived *Irg* genes

I established a cell culture-based system to explore the effect of wild rodents-derived *Irg*-like genes during *T. gondii* infection. For convenience, most xenogenous genes are expressed transiently. However, stable transfection is for several reasons preferred over transient transfection when a uniform population of host cells with a single copy of the introduced gene is desired. In transient transfection, the number of plasmid copies that enter the host cell could vary greatly, which creates noise and might lead to wrong interpretations of readouts. Additionally, the short recovery time between transient transfection of cells and their use in experiments might lead to cell stress influencing the phenotype (159). Thus, despite being a more tedious procedure, stable transfection is to be preferred when possible. We opted for the Flp-In cell system as the recipient for wild rodents-derived *Irg*-like genes. These cells allow stable expression of transgenic sequences in a reproducible manner (159). Commercially available parental strains contain a Flp Recombination Target (FRT) sequence which is recognized by a flipase (Flp) recombinase allowing a site-specific integration of genes of interest. The latter requires a cloning step in a plasmid containing a FRT site, to allow insertion of the gene. Parental cells are isogenic, meaning they have the same genetic background. This feature allows a streamlined creation of clonal cell lines avoiding the time-consuming single cell expansion step. However, despite being genetically identical, single cells within the isogenic population might have slightly different growth characteristics (148), thus single cell expansion might still be necessary. Within the possible Flp-In systems, Flp-In-3T3 was the cell line of choice since it is the only *M. musculus* cell line available. Furthermore, NIH/3T3 fibroblasts, which are the parental cells of Flp-In-3T3, are referred to as highly transfectable cells, which is a crucial aspect for molecular cloning. As for *T. gondii* infection, fibroblasts are one the most studied cell types for *in vitro* studies and their cell-autonomous immune response is believed to be crucial for limiting parasite burden.

Flp-In-3T3 cells were confirmed to be of *M. musculus* species via sequencing of the *CytB* gene. NIH/3T3 are derived from embryonic fibroblasts of the inbred NIH Swiss strain and the *Irgb2-b1* genotype was confirmed to be identical to the published inbred sequences from Lilue et al. as expected (reported in Fig. 9, (7)). This is crucial since the introduced gene will be present in addition to the endogenous *Irgb2-b1*. We assume that since inbred *M. musculus*-derived cells are not able to control virulent parasite infection, an observed parasite control by Flp-In-3T3 cells transfected with a wild rodent *Irg*-like gene can be attributed to the introduced gene.

6.1.5.1 Establishment of suitable vectors for the cloning strategy

The expression system of choice requires the use of suitable vectors, for example containing a FRT site to mediate site-specific insertion of the gene. Additional features facilitate the identification of successfully transfected cells as well as the intracellular localization of the expressed xenogenous protein. For this reason, establishment of suitable vectors was a prerequisite for the setup.

For the introduction of *Irg*-like genes in Flp-In-3T3 cells we developed a cloning strategy with two different plasmids: pES51-bl and pFS-1 (Fig. 13). *Irg*-like genes were first introduced in the pES51-bl plasmid using the SLiCE cloning method. Amplification of *Irg*-like genes with SLiCE-adapted primers with overhangs encoding for recombinase sites allows cloning of the gene of interest in a single-step reaction (Fig. 13a). After confirmation of successful cloning by colony PCR and sequencing of the gene, the latter was transferred to the pFS-1 vector. This insertion was performed via Golden Gate Assembly system, which is a non classical cloning method ((137), and explained further in chapter 5.1.6). This cloning method is convenient for recombining genes of interest and has e.g. already been used to study pathogenicity-conferring components in bacteria (160). This system allows us for example to explore the resistance activity of different *Irgb2*-like genes, by combining different exons to identify the ones responsible for the resistant phenotype. The Golden Gate Assembly system is based on Type IIS endonucleases which cut out of the recognized sequence and leave sticky overhangs. This renders the method particularly useful for cloning purposes. We integrated the restriction SapI site (GCTCTTC1/4) in the SLiCE primers' overhangs for *Irg*-like amplification, which allowed us to clone genes in pFS-1 with the methionine as start codon and in frame with an HA-Tag at the carboxy-terminal. However, the adaptation of SapI sites at the C-terminal implied the loss of the last two amino acids before the stop codon of IRGb1-like proteins, visible in the alignment in Fig. 9. Both SLiCE and Golden Gate cloning methods were successful and always led to a majority of positive clones. However, Golden Gate recombination was complicated by the presence of a possible SapI site within the sequence, which indeed happened for cloning of tandem *Irg*-like sequences in chapter 6.1.5.4. Identification of full length sequences required a change in the assembly protocol by using suboptimal digestion parameters for temperature and time, as explained in Material and Methods in chapter 5.1.6. Successfully cloned plasmids were positively selected via CcdB protein toxicity (136).

Once wild rodents-derived sequences were cloned in the final vector pFS-1, they were introduced into the Flp-In-3T3 cell system, i.e. transfected. Transfected cells can be identified by the green fluorescent nucleus, since pFS-1 carries EGFP expressed with a nuclear localization signal (3xNLS, Fig. 13b). Expression of the cloned gene is regulated by the human elongation factor 1α (EF-1α) promoter which induces a strong and constitutive expression. Also, as anticipated the gene is in frame with a C-terminal HA-Tag, thus expression and intracellular localization of the protein can be determined. Co-transfection with the pOG44 plasmid encoding for the yeast-derived Flp recombinase allowed site-specific integration of the gene of interest via FRT sites present on both pFS-1 and in the Flp-In-3T3 genome (Fig. 13c). Stably integrated cells were selected via Hygromycin B treatment.

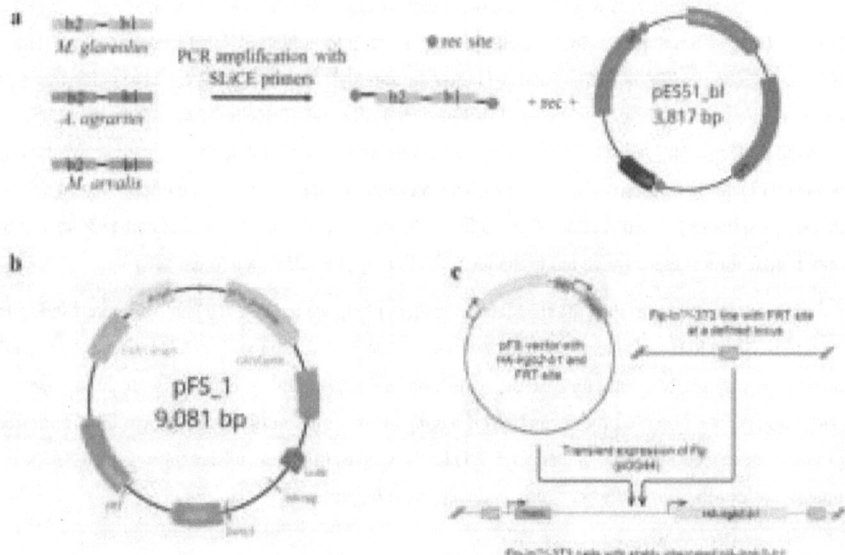

Fig. 13. Cloning strategy of *Irg*-like genes in Flp-In-3T3. In sequential order: (a) Cloning of *Irg*-like genes into pES51-bl via SLiCE cloning method. (b) pFS-1 vector where *Irg*-like genes are cloned from pES51-bl via Golden Gate assembly method. (c) Stable transfection of Flp-In-3T3 with pFS-1 carrying *Irg*-like genes. The last figure was modified from Niewiadomski and Rohatgi (148).

6.1.5.2 Establishment of the optimal transfection protocol for Flp-In-3T3 cells

Transfection in Flp-In-3T3 cells posed higher challenges than expected because of the size of pFS-1 (9,081 bp). The plasmid size increases further when a tandem *Irgb2-b1* gene is cloned in the vector, as for the positive control *Irgb2-b1*$_{CIM}$ sequence creating a final pFS-CIM plasmid 9,741bp-long. Here, the aim was to identify the protocol leading to the highest possible transient transfection rate in order to increase the probability to obtain stable transfected cells. For this purpose, different not viral-transfection methods and reagents were tested with both a commercially available pmaxGFP® and the pFS-CIM plasmids. More details about the reagents are reported in chapter 5.3.4.

Despite the reputation of NIH/3T3 cells to be highly suitable for transfection, not more than 20 % of the derived Flp-In-3T3 cells got transfected in my hands (Tab. 18). A higher transfection rate was observed when using small dimension plasmids, as the commercially available pmaxGFP® (3,486 bp) used to determine transfection efficiency, but decreased drastically when using pFS-CIM (Tab. 18). Transfection efficiency was estimated by the number of green fluorescent cells on the total of Hoechst 33342 stained nuclei on living cells 24 h after transfection. Unfortunately, despite many rounds of optimization and the use of a NIH/3T3-specific kit (*Amaxa*® *Cell Line Nucleofector Kit R*), the cost-efficient electroporation was not successful for pFS-CIM transfection. Combined with an extremely high mortality rate (> 95 %), positive clones were never identified (Tab. 18). The highest proportion of pmaxGFP®-transfected cells was observed when using Lipofectamine™3000 and *jetPRIME*®, 15 and 20 % respectively. The reported values are only slightly lower than published transfection rates on NIH/3T3 with Lipofectamine™2000 (161) and a similar lipid-based Attractene reagent (162). Interestingly, immunofluorescence assays of pFS-CIM-transfected Flp-In-3T3 cells with Lipofectamine™3000 detected a specific HA-tagged IRGb2-b1 signal in cells where the EGFP nuclear signal was weak or not detectable (Tab. 18 and visible in Fig. 14b). This resulted in a higher percentage of transfected cells by this staining than by sole detection of green fluorescent nuclei. However, Lipofectamine™3000 was the only transfection reagent which led to the identification of pFS-CIM-transfected cells.

Lipofectamine™ *3000* was then the transfection reagent of choice to clone the gene of interest in Flp-In-3T3 cells via pFS-1, and integration was possible via co-transfection with pOG44. The consequently higher amount of DNA used for stable transfection did not negatively interfere with the transfection rate, however we observed the formation of aggregates in solution (data not shown). The optimized protocol (described in details in chapter 5.3.4) leads reliably to the establishment of Flp-In-3T3 stable transfected cell lines in two weeks-time under constant Hygromycin B selection.

Tab. 18. Transfection methods and reagents tested on Flp-In-3T3 cells and the estimated transfection efficiency with either the control plasmid pmaxGFP* or pFS-CIM. Each reagent/protocol was tried at least twice. na = not assessed.

Reagent	Transfection efficiency (pmaxGFP®) [%]	pFS-CIM transfected cells [%]
25KDa linear Polyethylenimine (PEI)	5	0
PolyMag™	na	0
TransIT-X2®, TransIT-LT1® and TransIT-2020®	0	0
jetPRIME®	20	0 (0 % by HA-staining)
Amaxa® Cell Line Nucleofector Kit R	< 1	0
Lipofectamine™3000	15	1 (10 % by HA-staining Fig.14b)

6.1.5.3 Establishment of positive and negative control Flp-In-3T3 cell lines

At first I needed to validate the results of Lilue et al. in our expression system. I thus established positive and negative control cell lines by stably transfecting Flp-In-3T3 with the murine inbred *Irgb2-b1*$_{BL6}$ sequence, cloned in pFS-BL6, and the *M. musculus castaneus Irgb2-b1*$_{CIM}$ sequence, cloned in pFS-CIM, associated with susceptibility and resistance to virulent *T. gondii* respectively. After the establishment of a reliable protocol, the production of the two cell lines, named Flp-BL6 and Flp-CIM, was straightforward. Cell lines were confirmed to express the cloned *Irgb2-b1* genes via Western Blot of cell lysates with an anti-HA-tag antibody. As expected from the expression system, the amount of constitutively-expressed protein is equal in the created cell lines (Fig. 14a). Furthermore, I performed an immunofluorescence assay to investigate the intracellular localization of the protein. In uninfected cells IRGb2-b1 accumulates in reticular structures, similarly to what observed by Lilue et. al (Fig. 14b, (163)). During *T. gondii* infection of Flp-CIM cells, IRGb2-b1 relocates on the parasitophorous vacuole membrane (PVM) colocalizing with the parasite protein GRA7 (Fig. 14 b and c). GRA7 mediates ROP binding and phosphorylation of IRG proteins (164), is a useful staining for the PVM and differentiates between parasite's active invasion, where GRA7 is secreted and loaded on the PVM, from phagocytosis. These results also highlight that we underestimated the pFS-CIM transfection efficiency, since the EGFP nuclear signal is not always visible from cells that express the HA-tagged IRGb2-b1, thus obviously transfected (Fig. 14b). Importantly IRGb2-b1 loading is independent of IFN-γ treatment, also in accordance to what previously observed in resistant cell lines (163). These results confirm that in our expression system the positive and negative control proteins are equally expressed and behave similarly to what previously published.

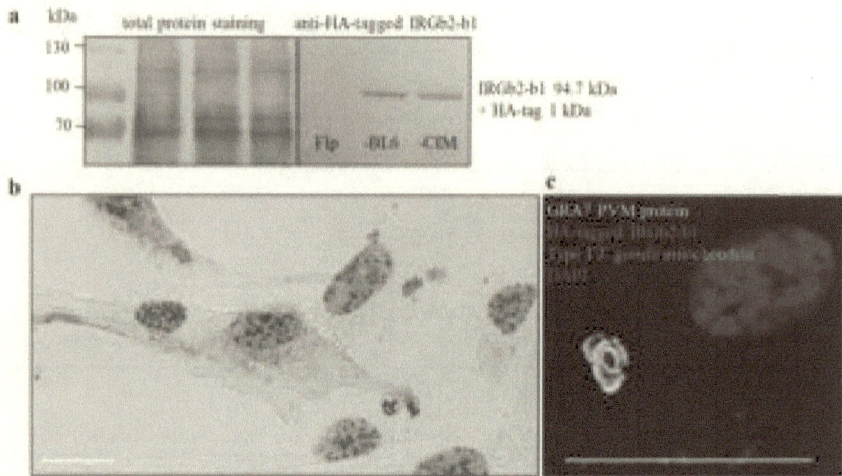

Fig. 14. The Flp-In-3T3-based system leads to comparable expression levels of transfected IRGb2-b1, which localizes on the PVM of virulent parasites. Flp-In-3T3 (Flp) parental strain was stably transfected with the negative (-BL6) and positive (-CIM) control *Irgb2-b1* gene, which is expressed in frame with an HA-tag. **(a)** DB71 total protein staining (left) and Western Blot with an anti-HA-tag antibody on the same membrane (right) of lysates from the three cell lines. First lane of the total protein staining with molecular weight marker (with sizes in kDa given to the left). A representative experiment of two replicates is shown. **(b, c)** Immunofluorescence assay of Flp-CIM cell line expressing an HA-tagged IRGb2-b1. Flp-CIM cells were infected for 1 h with a virulent *T. gondii* strain expressing a green fluorescent protein in the mitochondria, RHβGFPmt. In uninfected cells IRGb2-b1 accumulates in intracellular structures, whereas on *T. gondii* infected cells it relocates on the PVM (b) as shown by colocalizing with GRA7 (c). Following staining is shown: IRGb2-b1 (red), GRA7 (yellow), DAPI staining for nuclei (blue). A representative image is shown. The scale bar represents 20 μm.

6.1.5.4 Establishment of stable Flp-In-3T3 cell lines with wild rodents-derived *Irg*-like genes

Given the efficient and successful establishment of cell lines with the murine control sequences, I then proceeded with wild rodents-derived *Irg*-like sequences. I first transfected tandem *Irg*-like genes from the available wild rodents-derived cell lines, and in particular the identified tandem from *M. glareolus* BVK168 cells and tandem 1 from *A. agrarius* AAL-R cells (visible in Fig. 9). The cloning strategy used for *Irgb2-b1*~BL6~ and *Irgb2-b1*~CIM~ and explained in previous chapters was used to clone these wild rodents' sequences in pFS-1, resulting in pFS-BVK and pFS-AAL transfected in Flp-In-3T3 cells. Surprisingly, I observed an HA-tagged protein of 50 kDa instead of the expected 100 kDa, via Western Blot of cellular lysates from the created Flp-BVK and Flp-AAL cell lines (Fig. 15a). Nevertheless, these smaller IRG-like proteins loaded on the PVM of virulent parasites, as seen via immunofluorescent detection with an anti-HA-tag antibody (Fig 15b). I then PCR-amplified the full lenght genes from the plasmids used for cloning, to investigate the reason behind the detected smaller proteins. Full lenght genes were observed in pES51 cloned plasmids. However, pFS-BVK and pFS-AAL had a shorter inserted gene compared to positive control cells (Fig. 15c). A closer look to the full lenght sequences identified two additional SapI sites in both tandem *Irg*-like genes, the first exactly at the end of the *Irgb2*-like exon and the second 50 bp prior *Irgb1*-like C-terminal (Fig. 15d). Sequencing of both pFS-BVK and pFS-AAL plasmids confirmed sequence digestion at these sites during Golden Gate Assembly and ligation of the two fragments creating a shorter version of the gene with a gap of 1,256 bp in the *Irgb1*-like exon. The use of a reverse primer binding the *Irgb2*-like exon for colony PCR on cloned pFS plasmids did not allow identification of these truncated *Irg*-like sequences before establishment of the cell lines. However, this mistake allowed me to observe that the IRGb2-subunit only –together with the last residues of IRGb1– is sufficient for binding to the PVM of virulent parasites.

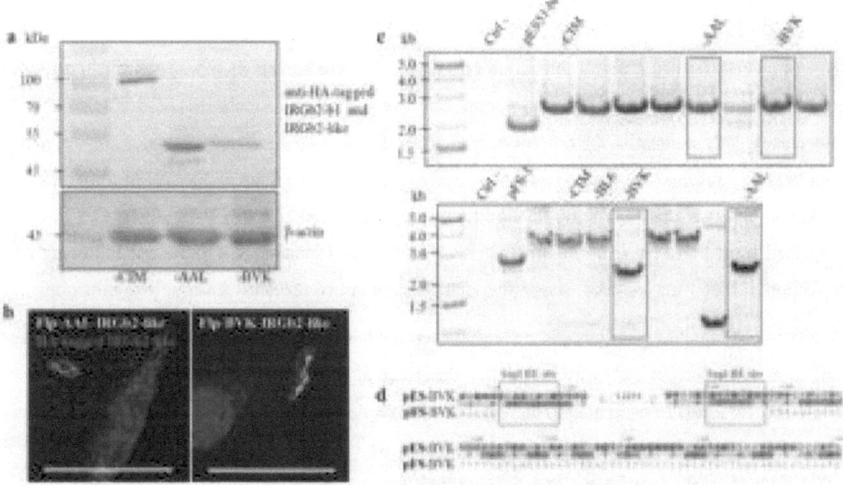

Fig. 15. The IRGb2 subunit is sufficient for binding to virulent parasites vacuole membranes. (a) DB71 total protein staining (left) and Western Blot (right) with an anti-HA-tag antibody. First lane with molecular weight marker (with sizes in kDa given to the left). A representative experiment of two replicates is shown. **(b)** Immunofluorescence assay of Flp-AAL-IRGb2-like cell line (left) and Flp-BVK-IRGb2-like cell line (right) expressing an HA-tagged IRGb2-b1. Cells were infected for 1 h with a virulent *T. gondii* strain expressing a green fluorescent protein in the mitochondria, RHβGFPmt.

Following staining is shown: IRGb2-b1 (red), *T. gondii* mitochondria (green), DAPI staining for nuclei (blue). A representative image is shown. The scale bar represents 20 μm. **(c)** 1 % agarose gels loaded with PCR-amplified *Irg* aand *Irg*-like tandem genes cloned in the pES51- bl plasmid (upper gel) and in the pFS-1 plasmid (lower gel). Red boxes highlight full length BVK and AAL sequences cloned in pES51- bl and truncated BVK and AAL sequences cloned in pFS-1. Positive and negative control sequences (-CIM and –BL6) and empty plasmids are indicated for comparison. First lane with DNA ladder (with sizes in kb given to the left). **(d)** Alignment of the full (pES-BVK) and truncated (pFS-BVK) versions of BVK *Irg*-like tandem genes. Red boxes highlight SapI sites within the sequence. Nucleotides positions relative to the full lenght sequence are reported above the sequences. Nucleotide sequences are reported, and for the full lenght pES-BVK also the translated sequence.

6.1.5.5 *T. gondii* infection phenotype in established positive and negative control cell lines

Host-mediated *T. gondii* killing is followed by programmed death of the cell itself (109). An association between this phenotype and host resistance was suggested, since the parasite niche gets disrupted (7, 150). On the contrary, susceptible cells allow parasite proliferation until active egress of the same around 48 hpi. Resistant *M. musculus castaneus* CIM cells display an IFN-γ-dependent increase in necrotic cell death for both type I and type II infection, whereas susceptible BL6 cells display this phenotype only following avirulent infection (7). I will then refer to the IFN-γ-mediated cell death as the resistance phenotype.

Necrotic death results in permeabilization of both plasma and nuclear membranes. I thus performed a double staining with both a nuclear impermeable dye, Propidium Iodide (PI), and a permeable one, Hoechst 33342, to quantify the ratio of necrotic cells during *T. gondii* infection and IFN-γ stimulation, similarly to published protocols (150). As shown in Fig. 16, an increase in necrotic murine Flp-In-3T3 cells was observed during type II infection following stimulation with IFN-γ, however not to the extent expected from literature (7). A similar increase in PI⁺ cells increase was observed following type I infection of IFN-γ-treated cells, suggesting that cells are not completely susceptible to infection.

We expected Flp-CIM positive cells to show an increase in necrotic cell death following IFN-γ treatment and *T. gondii* infection. Surprisingly, a rather decreased amount of necrotic cells was observed for both Flp-CIM and Flp-BL6 compared to the wild-type (wt) cell line (Fig. 16). No obvious control of parasite proliferation was observed at the microscope in positive control Flp-CIM cells compared to other cell lines. Indeed, preliminary experiments confirmed that IFN-γ treated Flp-CIM cells did not display a reduced number of parasites per vacuole compared to Flp-BL6 cells (Appendix Fig. 38).

Results suggest that our cell culture-based system does not reproduce results published in literature. Despite the identical *Irgb2-b1* genotype, Flp-In-3T3 cells display a different phenotype during *T. gondii* infection compared to other inbred mouse cells. A difference between the derived positive Flp-CIM and negative control Flp-BL6 cell lines is not obvious in regard to *T. gondii* infection.

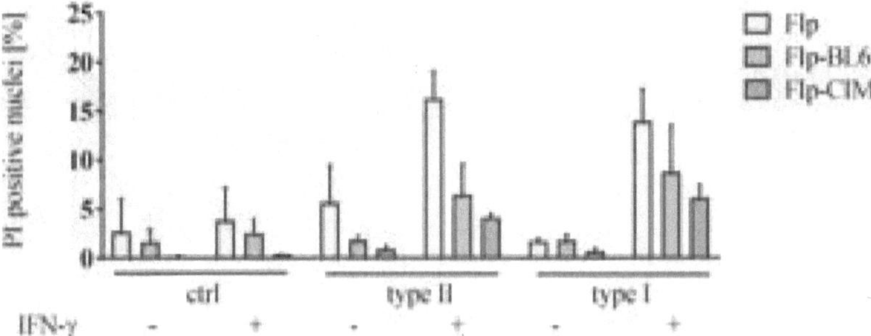

Fig. 16. The positive control cell line Flp-CIM does not display the host resistance phenotype. Flp-In-3T3 (Flp) parental strain, negative control Flp-BL6 and positive control Flp-CIM cell lines were treated with 200 U/ml mouse IFN- γ or left untreated 24 h prior infection with avirulent (type II) and virulent (type I) *T. gondii*. 24 hpi a double staining with Propidium Iodide (PI) and Hoechst 33342 on living cells was performed. Double stained nuclei were quantified at the fluorescent microscope. Mean ± sd (n = 3 experiments, each with 2 replicates).

6.1.5.6 Flp-In-3T3 cells express higher levels of endogenous *Irgb2-b1* compared to primary fibroblasts

The resistant phenotype described in CIM cells is influenced by polymorphisms in *Irg* sequences, but also by expression levels of the same (163). Surprisingly, the amount of endogenous IRGb2-b1 protein (indicated with a black arrow-head in Fig. 17a) in Flp-In-3T3 cells was higher than the introduced one (indicated with a red arrow-head), as observed via Western Blot with the anti-IRGb2-b1 serum. The observed IRGb2-b1 protein levels in Flp-In-3T3 cells were higher than in primary murine fibroblasts in literature (7). Thus, I established a primary murine fibroblasts culture to confirm its lower amount of IRGb2-b1 protein compared to immortalized murine Flp-In-3T3 cells.

Primary fibroblasts cultures were easily established from tails of inbred mice as explained in chapter 5.3.2. As expected, cells were susceptible to treatment with mouse IFN-γ, as shown by phosphorylation and nuclear translocation of STAT1 following treatment (Fig. 17b). Confirming our hypothesis, a strikingly lower IFN-γ-induced expression of IRGb2-b1 in primary fibroblasts than in Flp-In-3T3 cells was observed by Western Blot (Fig. 17c, (7)). However, the transcript abundance was only slightly lower in primary cells compared immortalized murine cells available to us (Fig. 17d). My results indicate a higher amount of endogenous IFN-γ-induced IRGb2-b1 in immortalized fibroblast cell lines compared to primary cultures.

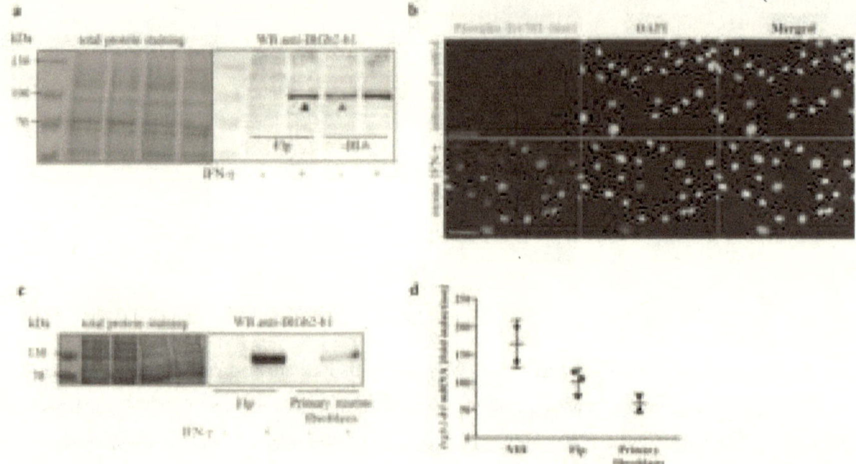

Fig. 17. Flp-In-3T3 cells express high level of endogenous IRGb2-b1 compared to primary murine fibroblasts. (a) DB71 total protein staining (left) and Western Blot with anti-IRGb2-b1 serum on the same membrane (right) of lysates from Flp-In-3T3 and Flp-BL6 cells. Cells were treated for 24 h with mouse IFN-γ (200 U/ml) or left untreated as control. The black arrow-head indicates the endogenous IRGb2-b1 protein in Flp-In-3T3 parental cells, and the red arrow-head the xenogenous IRGb2-b1$_{BL6}$ in Flp-BL6 cells. First lane with molecular weight marker (with sizes in kDa given to the left). A representative experiment of three replicates is shown. **(b)** Established primary murine fibroblast cell cultures are responsive to mouse IFN-γ (200 U/ml). In each panel the following stainings are shown from left to right: phospho-Tyr701-STAT1 staining (green), DAPI staining (white) and overlay of the two signals. Activated phospho-STAT1 is indicated by nuclear translocation. A representative experiment of two replicates is shown. The scale bar represents 50 μm. **(c)** DB71 total protein staining (left) and Western Blot with anti-IRGb2-b1 serum on the same membrane (right) of lysates from Flp-In-3T3 and primary murine fibroblasts. Cells were treated for 24 h with mouse IFN-γ (200 U/ml) or left untreated as control. First lane with molecular weight marker (with sizes in kDa given to the left). A representative experiment of two replicates is shown. **(d)** *Irgb2-b1* mRNA abundance in primary murine fibroblasts is lower than in NIH/3T3 cells and almost equal to Flp-In-3T3 cells. Cells were treated for 24 h with either treated with mouse IFN-γ (200 ng/ml) or left untreated as control. The reported mRNA fold induction is relative to untreated cells (set as 1; not shown) and normalised to Ywhaz for reference. Each point indicates a biological replicate, each with two technical replicates.

6.1.5.7 The endogenous *Irgb2-b1* does not interfere with the transfected gene in Flp-In-3T3 cells

Results indicate that Flp-In-3T3 cells express a higher amount of endogenous IRGb2-b1 compared to the introduced protein and to primary cell lines susceptible to *T. gondii* infection. We speculated that loading on the PVM of an eccessive amount of a not susceptible protein might interfere with the infection phenotype in our Flp-based system. To validate this hypothesis, we knock-out (KO) the endogenous *Irgb2-b1* from Flp-In-3T3 cells. The resulting Flp Δb2b1 line was used to establish new stable positive and negative control cell lines, i.e. Flp Δb2b1-CIM and Flp Δb2b1-BL6.

The KO was performed by Tobias Steinfeldt (University of Freiburg, Germany) via CRISPR-Cas9 with a recently published protocol (115). I clonally amplified several clones from the resulting pool of KO cells to identify a clonal cell line lacking both copies of the allele. I identified one suitable clone, named Flp Δb2b1 and indicated in the red box in Fig. 18a, by Western Blot with the anti-IRGb2-b1 serum. The correspondent lane lacks the band at ~100 KDa, similarly to the negative control CIM *Irgb2-b1* KO cells (CIM Δb2b1, (115)). KO of *Irgb2-b1* from Flp-In-3T3 cells was further confirmed via RT-qPCR (data not shown). The faint band with similar size present in all lanes, and particularly visible for KO cells, is likely another IRG tandem protein recognized by the anti-IRGb2-b1 serum. Indeed, the peptide sequence at the protein C-terminal used to develop the serum is conserved amongs tandem IRGs (7).

Flp Δb2b1 was used for cloning of *Irgb2-b1*[BL6] and *Irgb2-b1*[CIM], as already performed with the wt cell line, resulting in positive Flp Δb2b1-CIM and negative Flp Δb2b1-BL6 control cell lines. I performed a PI-assay to evaluate the phenotype of the newly established cell lines to infection with *T. gondii*. The three cell lines – i.e. Flp Δb2b1, Flp Δb2b1-CIM and Flp Δb2b1-BL6 – display the same phenotype to infection with type I and II T. gondii, with and without IFN-γ treatment (Fig. 18b). Notably, I did not observe an increase of necrotic cell death in IFN-γ-treated Flp Δb2b1-CIM cells following parasite infection. Data rather suggest an opposite trend, similarly to what observed for wt Flp-In-3T3 clones (Fig. 16). Furthermore, cells did not exhibit striking differences in parasite burden as observed at the microscope (data not shown).

The developed cell culture-based system does not replicate results from literature despite Flp-In-3T3 cells carry the *Irgb2-b1* susceptible allele. The gene is more expressed compared to other murine fibroblast cultures. However, we showed here that the higher amount of endogenous IRGb2-b1 is not responsible for the lack of reproducibilty of published phenotypes in the Flp-based system. Taken together, our results indicate that the Flp-In-3T3 cells cannot be used to study the *Irg*-like-mediated resistance to T. gondii.

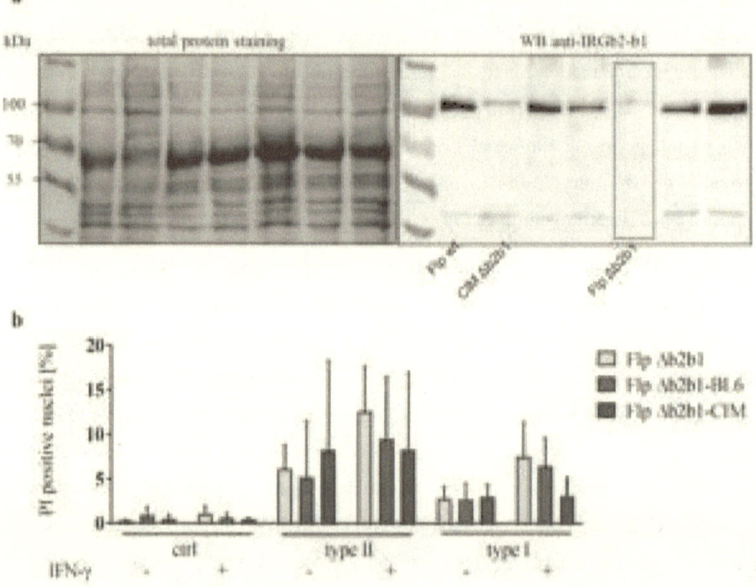

Fig. 18. The endogenous IRGb2-b1 protein in Flp-In-3T3 cells does not interfere with the resistance phenotype of IRGb2-b1$_{\text{CIM}}$**.** *Irgb2-b1* was knock-out from Flp-In-3T3 cells via CRISPR-Cas9 and resulting clonal cell line was stably transfected with resistance-associated *Irgb2-b1*$_{\text{CIM}}$ and susceptibility-associated *Irgb2-b1*$_{\text{BL6}}$. **(a)** DB71 total protein staining (left) and Western Blot (right) with an anti-IRGb2-b1 serum. Flp-In-3T3 wt (Flp wt), the negative control CIM *Irgb2-b1* KO cells (CIM Δb2b1) and different clonal cell lines established from Flp-In-3T3 *Irgb2-b1* KO cells were treated for 24 h with mouse IFN-γ (200 U/ml). Identified *Irgb2-b1* KO cell line (Flp Δb2b1) is highlighted by the red box. First lane with molecular weight marker (with sizes in kDa given to the left). A representative experiment of two replicates is shown. **(b)** Established Flp ΔIrgb2b1, Flp ΔIrgb2b1-CIM and Flp ΔIrgb2b1-BL6 cell lines were treated with 200 U/ml mouse IFN-γ or left untreated 24 h prior infection with avirulent (type II) and virulent (type I) *T. gondii*. 24 hpi a double staining with Propidium Iodide (PI) and Hoechst 33342 on living cells was performed and double stained nuclei were quantified at the fluorescent microscope. Mean ± sd (n = 2 experiments, each with 2 replicates).

6.2 Production of recombinant *M. glareolus* IFN-γ

Results from the following chapter have been published on my first author paper Torelli et al. (124). Figures and a limited number of sentences in this result section (chapter 6.2) as well as the relative discussion (chapter 7.3.1) have been left unchanged from the published manuscript.

6.2.1 Limited sequence conservation of IFN-γ between different rodent species

The availability of *M. glareolus*-derived cell systems allowed us to study vole cells' susceptibility to *T. gondii* infection. Because of our interest in IFN-γ-induced *Irg* genes and the central role of the cytokine during infection, access to an active type II interferon on *M. glareolus* cells was a prerequisite for the project. Diversity in the protein sequence of IFN-γ results in species-specific activity of the cytokine (165). We compared available IFN-γ genomic sequences of various rodents to predict cross-reactivity of the commercially available murine cytokine on vole-derives cell cultures. *Peromyscus maniculatus* and *H. sapiens* were used as more distant species for comparison (Fig. 19a).

Amino acid sequences within the Arvicolinae cluster species – i.e. *Microtus ochrogaster*, *M. agrestis*, *Ellobius lutescens* and *M. glareolus* – and within the Murinae cluster species – i.e. *M. musculus*, *A. sylvaticus* and *R. norvegicus* – share more than 83 % sequence identity over the entire sequence (Fig. 19a). In contrast, there is a high divergence between murid and arvicoline clusters, with *M. musculus* and *M. glareolus* sharing only 57.3 % amino acid sequence identity.

Core regions of the protein (underlined areas in Fig. 19b) have a high sequence conservation between species, whereas the rest of the IFN-γ sequence is less conserved out of the same phylogenetic clade. In particular, certain residues previously implicated in the binding of IFN-γ with the receptor (IFN-γR1) (165) have a high degree of sequence divergence between murid and cricetid rodents (red boxes in Fig. 19b). The basic lysine and arginine-rich stretch, located at the C-terminal end of murine IFN-γ (Fig. 19b; "basic stretch"), is highly conserved in all IFN-γ sequences and has also been implicated in receptor binding (165, 166). After the basic stretch, a C-terminal extension of the IFN-γ sequence is present in cricetid rodents but not in murine species, whereas present but divergent in the human homologue gene (Fig. 19b). Taken together, there is low sequence conservation between murid and cricetid sequences and we anticipated that the commercial mouse IFN-γ would not be active on vole cells.

Fig. 19 (following page). Protein sequence diversity of IFN-γ within rodent species. (a) Amino acid sequence similarity (in percentage) of IFN-γ proteins. On the left, a dendrogram based on IFN-γ sequence similarity is shown, whereby *Peromyscus maniculatus* and *H. sapiens* served as more distant species for comparison. The Arvicolinae (red branches) and the Murinae species (blue branches) are indicated. **(b)** IFN-γ amino acid sequence comparison between different rodent species and *H. sapiens*. Light blue indicates lower percentage of identity than dark blue. Arrow head indicates the *M. musculus* signal peptide cleavage site. Residues involved in the binding to the receptor subunit IFN-γR1 are highlighted by red boxes. Functionally important regions and the C-terminal basic domain are indicated (165). Both figures were created by Frank Seeber (Robert Koch-Institut).

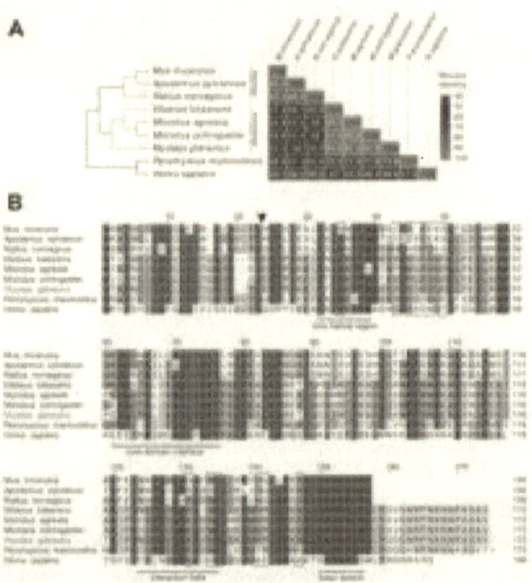

6.2.2 Production of recombinant M. glareolus IFN-γ in E. coli

Given the expected lack of activity of the murine IFN-γ on vole cells, heterologous expression of *M. glareolus* recombinant IFN-γ (recMgIFN-γ) was performed in *Escherichia coli* OmniMax 2T1R cells. The deposited *Mg*IFN-γ sequence (GenBank HQ650825) was cloned in frame with a C-terminal 6His-tag into a tetracycline-regulated expression vector, resulting in the created plasmid pASG33-*Mg*IFN-γ. Rec*Mg*IFN-γ expression was robust, yielding generally >3 mg/l of soluble protein after a single round of purification by immobilised metal affinity chromatography. SDS-PAGE analysis of the purified protein showed three major bands (20, 42 and 65 kDa; inferred from a standard curve based on the molecular weight (MW) markers) and two minor bands (15 and >100 kDa; Fig. 20a). The four largest proteins reacted with an anti-6His antibody and are interpreted as monomer, dimer, trimer and higher order aggregates. Their molecular masses are in good agreement with the calculated MW of monomeric rec*Mg*IFN-γ containing a 6His-tag (18.3 kDa). Rec*Mg*IFN-γ production in *E. coli* and its analysis via Western Blot were performed by Florian Müller (Robert Koch Institut). I tested the cross-reactivity of a commercial anti-human IFN-γ antibody on rec*Mg*IFN-γ by Western Blot. However, given the great diversity of IFN-γ sequences, especially of the tagged epitope in position 31-80 (Fig. 19b), the antibody did not cross-react as expected (data not shown).

Since IFN-γ needs to be in a homodimeric form to activate its receptor, the purified rec*Mg*IFN-γ was analysed by gel filtration by Frank Seeber (Robert Koch-Institut). This analysis determines the proportion of different protein aggregates in the preparations. As shown in Fig. 20b, the vast majority of the applied protein eluted at a column volume which is consistent with the dimeric form (36.4 kDa observed vs. 36.6 kDa calculated).

Since lipopolysaccharide (LPS) of bacterial origin can induce *Irg* expression in murine macrophages (167), another recombinant protein was produced in the same *E. coli* strain to exclude an aspecific activity of bacteria fragments in the rec*Mg*IFN-γ preparation. Therefore, *T. gondii* Late Embryogenesis Abundant (LEA) 870 protein (Gene ID TGME49_076870) was cloned in plasmid pQE90S in frame with a 6His-tag, and expressed similarly to rec*Mg*IFN-γ in OmniMax 2T1R. Recombinant Rec*Tg*LEA production was performed by Sandra Klein (Robert Koch-Institut). As expected, Rec*Tg*LEA was expressed as monomeric protein of 17.9 KDa, similar in mass to rec*Mg*IFN-γ (personal communication from Benedikt Fabian, Robert Koch-Institut).

Collectively, these results show that a single affinity chromatography purification of recMgIFN-γ resulted in a large proportion of soluble, dimeric and thus presumably correctly folded and active protein. Another recombinant protein produced in the same bacteria strain allows us to test for the specific activity of recMgIFN-γ, especially in the context of *Irg* genes induction.

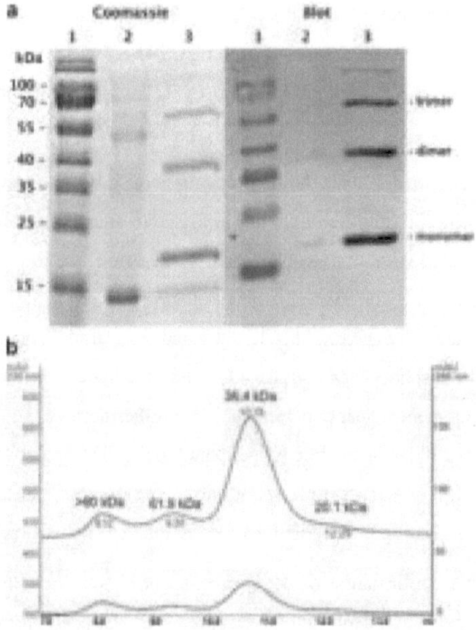

Fig. 20. rec*Mg*IFN-γ purified by immobilised metal affinity chromatograph is mostly in a dimeric form. (a) SDS-PAGE followed by Coomassie staining for total protein detection (left) and detection of 6His-tagged proteins by Western Blot with an anti-6His monoclonal antibody (right). Lane 1: molecular weight marker (with sizes in kDa given to the left - sizes greater than 100 kDa were unreliable when constructing a standard curve); lane 2: flow-through (unbound proteins); lane 3: purified protein(s). SDS-PAGE and Western Blot performed by Florian Müller (Robert Koch-Institut). **(b)** Size determination of purified rec*Mg*IFN-γ by analytical gel filtration analysis on a pre-calibrated Superdex

75 column. Protein peaks were detected at 230 nm (red) and 260 nm (blue), respectively. The gel filtration analysis was performed by Frank Seeber (Robert Koch-Institut).

6.2.3 rec*Mg*IFN-γ activates STAT1 signaling in vole cell lines

When IFN-γ activates its signaling pathway, phosphorylation of cytosolic STAT1 at the residues Tyr701 and Ser727 and its subsequent nuclear translocation is observed. STAT1 is divergent between taxa; it shares the highest degree of homology within the DNA binding site and the lowest in the transactivation domain (168). The latter implies species-specific differences in interaction with cofactors involved in the IFN-γ pathway activation (169). However, STAT1 sequences from different species share conserved residues around the activating Tyr701 and Ser727. Thus, we anticipated that antibodies raised against the phosphorylated murine Tyr701-STAT1 and Tyr727-STAT1 proteins will cross-react on other rodent species.

I tested rec*Mg*IFN-γ activity on the already introduced vole-derived cell lines, the *M. glareolus* BVK168 and the *M. arvalis* FMN-R cell lines. Mouse IFN-γ cross-reactivity was instead tested on *A. agrestis* AAL-R cells and used as positive control on *M. musculus* NIH/3T3 embryonic fibroblasts cell line. I therefore assessed co-localization of phosphorylated STAT1 with cell nuclei of treated cells by immunofluorescent assay (IFA) with an anti-phospho Tyr701-STAT1 antibody (similar to a previous study on bank vole cells (170)) and an anti-phospho Tyr727-STAT1 antibody on the mentioned cell lines.

M. musculus NIH/3T3 cells treated with the homologous mouse IFN-γ showed nuclear-localised and phosphorylated Tyr701-STAT1 (middle panel in Fig. 21). No signal was detected in either untreated NIH/3T3 cells or cells treated with rec*Mg*IFN-γ. As expected from the low IFN-γ sequence similarity between murine and vole species, following treatment of the *M. glareolus* BVK168 cell line with mouse IFN-γ we observed no nuclear signal, similarly in untreated cells (middle panel in Fig. 21). In contrast, a clear co-localization of phosphorylated Tyr701-STAT1 and cell nuclei was detected in BVK168 cells following rec*Mg*IFN-γ treatment (upper panel in Fig. 21). Furthermore, rec*Mg*IFN-γ but not mouse IFN-γ was active on a *M. arvalis* FMN-R cell line (upper panel in Fig. 21). Moreover, in the AAL-R cell line from *A. agrarius* mouse IFN-γ activated phosphorylation and nuclear translocation of STAT1 in this related murine species, confirming our predictions from sequence analysis (middle panel in Fig. 21).

The results gave us a first confirmation of the species-specific activity of rec*Mg*IFN-γ on bank vole cells, which are not responsive to the mouse IFN-γ as predicted. Rec*Mg*IFN-γ shows also activity on the *M. arvalis* cell line FMN-R, whereas the mouse IFN-γ is active on striped field mouse cells.

Fig. 21 (following page). Species-specific activity of rec*Mg*IFN-γ and mouse IFN-γ on different rodent cell lines. NIH/3T3, BVK168, FMN-R and AAL-R cells were tested and either left untreated as control (lower panel), stimulated for 1h with rec*Mg*IFN-γ (200 ng/ml, upper panel) or mouse IFN-γ (200 U/ml, central panel). In each panel the following stainings are shown from left to right: phospho-Tyr701-STAT1 staining (green), DAPI staining (white) and overlay of the two signals. Activated Phospho-STAT1 is indicated by nuclear translocation. A representative experiment of three replicates is shown. The scale bar represents 50 μm.

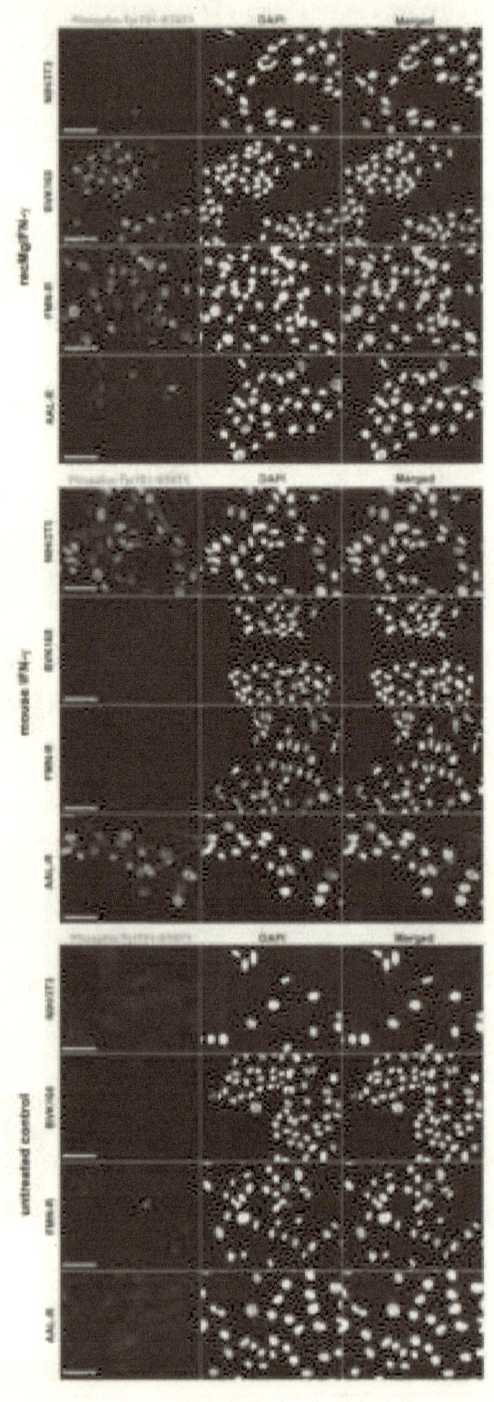

STAT1 activation persists longer than in other STAT isoforms (171). I confirmed that the IFN-γ-induced phosphorylation of STAT1 is not only detected 1 h post treatment (Fig. 21), but also at 24 h (Fig. 22) which is the time point of choice for the infection experiments in this project. Both STAT1 isoforms – i.e. STAT1a of 91 kDa and the C-terminal truncated version STAT1b of 84 kDa – are recognized by the anti-murine phospho-Tyr701-STAT1 antibody in both the murine Flp-In-3T3 cell line and in bank vole BVK168 cells 24 h after treatment with the respective IFN-γ (higher panel Fig. 22). Results suggest a higher phosphorylation level of the more transcriptionally active STAT1a isoform in the vole cell line compared to the murine one. The not phosphorylated form of STAT1 is highly induced following IFN-γ treatment in both cell lines as expected (Interferome REF, middle panel Fig. 22), in a higher degree in the murine cells compared to voles. However, the not phosphorylated form of STAT1 expected in untreated and LEA-treated controls was surprisingly not or barely detected at this time point (middle panel Fig. 22).

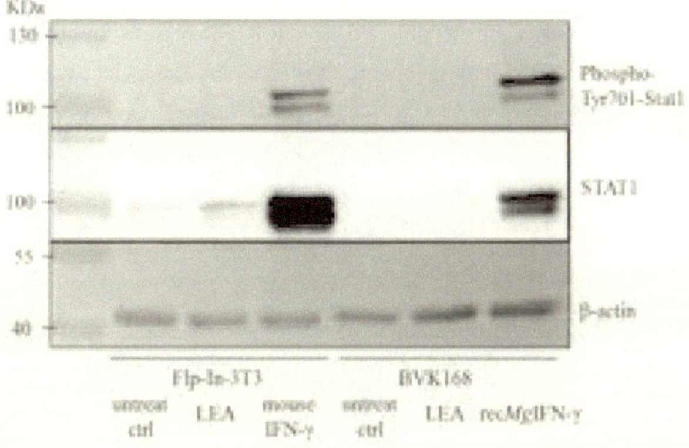

Fig. 22. STAT1 pathway is activated in BVK168 cells 24 h post treatment. Western Blot with anti-murine antibodies against phospho-Tyr701-STAT1 (upper panel), STAT1 (central panel) and β-actin (lower panel). Cells were treated for 24 h with either the negative control protein rec*Tg*LEA (LEA, 200 ng/ml), mouse IFN-γ (for Flp-In-3T3, 200 U/ml) or rec*Mg*IFN-γ (for BVK168, 200 ng/ml), or left untreated as control (untreat ctrl). A representative experiment of two replicates is shown. First lane with molecular weight marker (with sizes in kDa given to the left).

Since full transcriptional activity of STAT1a also requires Ser727 being phosphorylated (80), I assessed its phosphorylation status by an anti-mouse phospho-Ser727-STAT1 antibody in NIH/3T3, BVK168 and AAL-R cell lines. Via immunofluorescence assays I detected basal phosphorylation levels of Ser727 in all three cell lines, which reflects results already reported in literature (86). However, a clear increase in the nuclear signal correspondent to phospho-Ser727-STAT1 is obvious following treatment of BVK168 with rec*Mg*IFN-γ and AAL-R with the murine IFN-γ compared to untreated control cells (Fig.

23). These results mirror what observed for the residue Tyr701 and confirmed Ser727 of STAT1 being also phosphorylated.

Taken together, these results confirmed via different assays the species-specific activity of the produced recMgIFN-γ on *M. glareolus* BVK168 cells and *M. arvalis* FMN-R cells. Pathway activation induces the phosphorylation at the STAT1 activating residues Tyr701 and Tyr727. Furthermore, results show activity of the murine IFN-γ on *A. agrarius* AAL-R cells, confirming the prediction based on sequence identity with the murine cytokine. The IFN-γ pathway is activated not only one hour following treatment, but also 24 h later, which corresponds to the time point for *T. gondii* infection experiments.

Fig. 23 (following page). Ser727-STAT1 phosphorylation confirms the activity of recMgIFN-γ on BVK168 cell line and of mouse IFN-γ on AAL-R cell line. NIH/3T3, BVK168 and AAL-R were either stimulated for 1 h with recMgIFN-γ (200 ng/ml, upper panel), with mouse IFN-γ (200 U/ml, central panel) or left untreated as control (lower panel). In each panel the following staining is shown from left to right: phospho-Ser727-STAT1 staining (green), DAPI staining for nuclei (white) and overlay of the two signals. Activated Phospho-STAT1 is indicated by nuclear translocation. A representative experiment of two replicates is shown. The scale bar represents 100 μm.

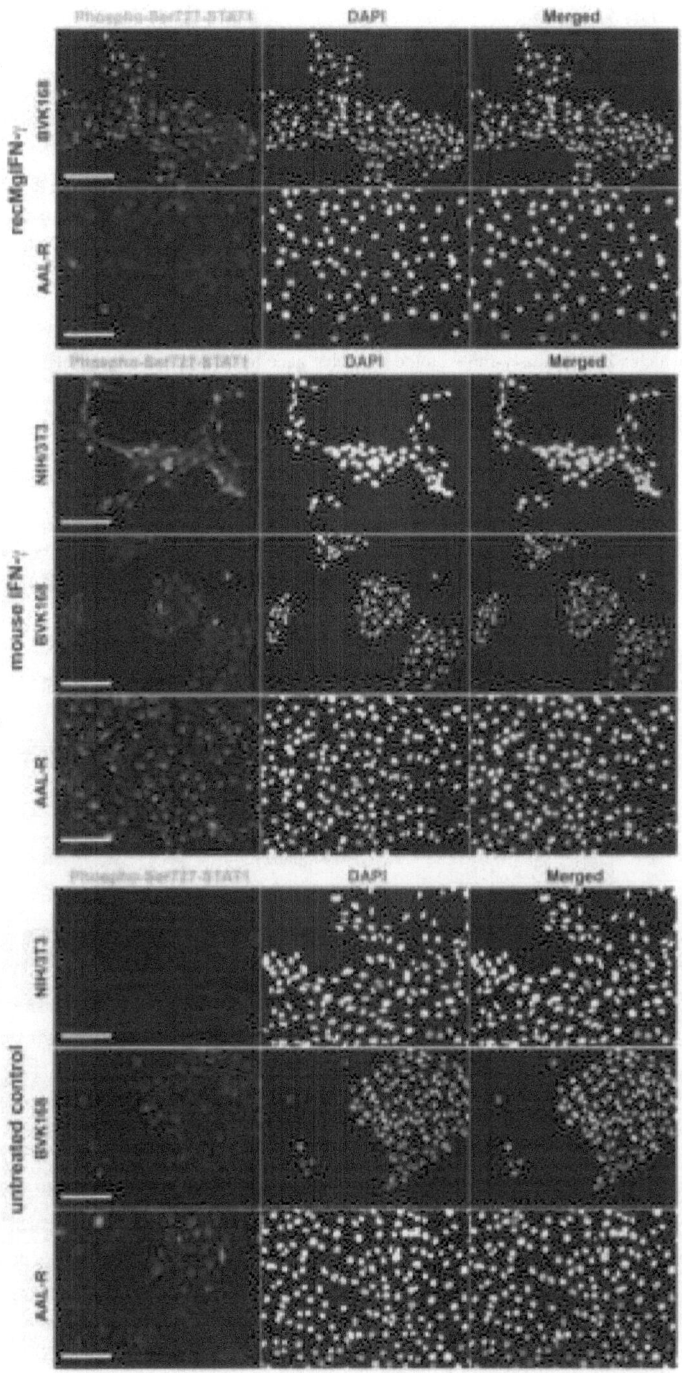

recMgIFNγ
Phospho-Ser727-STAT1
DAPI
Merged
BVK168
AAL-R
mouse IFNγ
Phospho-Ser727-STAT1
DAPI
Merged
NIH3T3
BVK168
AAL-R
untreated control
Phospho-Ser727-STAT1
DAPI
Merged
NIH3T3
BVK168
AAL-R

IFN-γ pathway activation leads to STAT1-mediated expression of numerous target genes, such as the *Irg* gene family in rodents. Due to our interest in this innate immune response gene family during infection with *T. gondii*, I measured the increase of mRNA of one of its members and our main focus, *Irgb2-b1*, by real-time quantitative Reverse Transcription PCR (qRT-PCR) as a further proof of rec*Mg*IFN-γ activity. At the same time I could assess the relative expression of this gene in the vole-derived cell lines BVK168 and FMN-R. I compared *Irgb2-b1* expression in cells treated with either rec*Mg*IFN-γ, murine IFN-γ, rec*Tg*LEA, or left untreated as control. As reference gene for normalization I used the tyrosine 3-monooxygenase/tryptophan 5-monooxygenase activation protein zeta gene (*Ywhaz*), which was previously shown to be a reliable gene for this purpose in the closely related field vole *M. agrestis* (134). Following rec*Mg*IFN-γ treatment, a dose-dependent relative increase in *Irgb2-b1* mRNA levels in both vole cell lines was observed, which reached 8-fold when 200 ng/ml protein was used, compared to untreated cells or cells treated with the control protein rec*Tg*LEA (Fig. 24). The latter confirmed a rec*Mg*IFN-γ-specific effect on this target gene rather than a non-specific cellular stimulation by bacterial contaminants. Taken together, these data demonstrated that rec*Mg*IFN-γ was capable of activating IFN-γ-dependent cellular responses in two cell lines of the two related vole species. However, in the same assay mouse IFN-γ was not active, corroborating the necessity for vole-specific IFN-γ.

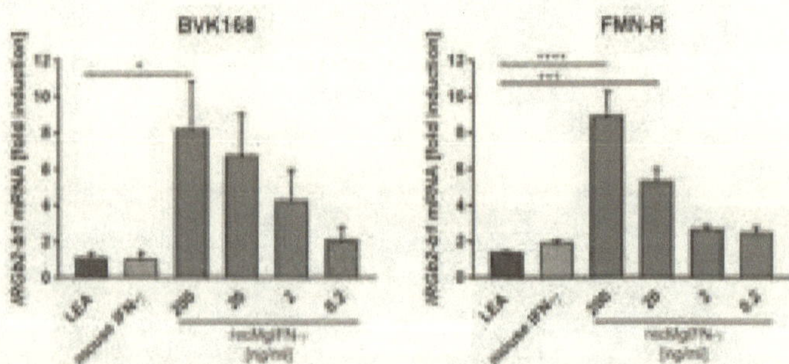

Fig. 24. Dose-dependent induction of the expression of the target gene *Irgb2-b1* by rec*Mg*IFN-γ in BVK168 and FMN-R cells. Bank vole BVK168 and common vole FMN-R cells were treated for 24 h with either the negative control protein LEA (200 ng/ml), mouse IFN-γ (200 U/ml) or recMgIFN-γ (10-fold dilution from 200 to 0.2 ng/ml). The reported mRNA fold induction is relative to untreated cells (set as 1; not shown) and normalised to *Ywhaz* for reference. Mean ± SEM (n = 3 experiments, each with 2 replicates) are shown. Statistical analysis: One-way Anova followed by Dunnett's multiple comparisons test (all against the LEA control protein). BVK168 (F(5,12) = 3.75, p=0.0282) * p=0.0322, FMN-R (F(5,12) = 21.34, p<0.0001) **** p= 0.0001, *** p=0.0004. Note that only statistically significant (p≤0.05) differences were depicted in the figure.

   rec*Mg*IFN-γ limits replication of vesicular stomatitis virus in bank vole cells

Testing for antiviral activity is a standard procedure for reporting biological activity of IFN-γ. BVK168 cells were previously shown to be permissive for a number of viruses including vesicular stomatitis virus (VSV) (125) known to be highly susceptible to IFN-γ treatment in murine cells (172, 173). Bank voles are known reservoir of murid herpesvirus (174, 175) also responding to the type II interferon response (176). Georg Kochs (University Freiburg, Germany) performed viral infections of BVK168 cells treated or not with rec*Mg*IFN-γ to test its antiviral activity. He used two luciferase expressing viral strains, as the VSV replicon VSV*ΔG(FLuc) (145) and a murine gammaherpesvirus 68 (MHV68), as an easy to follow reporter via bioluminescence readout for measuring the IFN-γ effect on virus replication. As positive control he used a human hybrid type I interferon, IFN-αB/D, shown previously to be active on a wide variety of mammalian species and to inhibit VSV virus replication (144), and as negative control rec*Tg*LEA to assess specificity of recMgIFN-γ. As shown in Fig. 25, we observed a drastic reduction of virus replication in VSV-infected BVK168 cells treated with 1 ng/ml recMgIFN-γ and to a lesser extent with a lower concentration (0.2 ng/ml). No obvious antiviral effect was seen in cells treated with the control protein LEA. These results demonstrate that rec*Mg*IFN-γ possesses antiviral activity using this host-virus system. However, rec*Mg*IFN-γ antiviral potency led to inconsistent results on MHV68-infected BVK168 cells (Fig. 25).

Vole BVK168 cells also proved to be susceptible to infection with cowpox virus (CXPV) isolates from both a Brazilian rodent (125) and from the closely related *M. arvalis* (177). In collaboration with Heinz Ellerbrok (Robert Koch-Institut), we infected BVK168 cells with a cowpox virus (CXPV) Brighton Red strain expressing a green fluorescent protein to further prove rec*Mg*IFN-γ antiviral capacity, given the dependancy of the virus on this pathway (178). Fluorescence detection is a convenient read-out for viral growth and equally sensitive to virus-related bioluminescence signal (173). Unfortunately, results on rec*Mg*IFN-γ-mediated control of CXPV Brighton Red strain replication in BVK168 cells were inconsistent (data not shown).

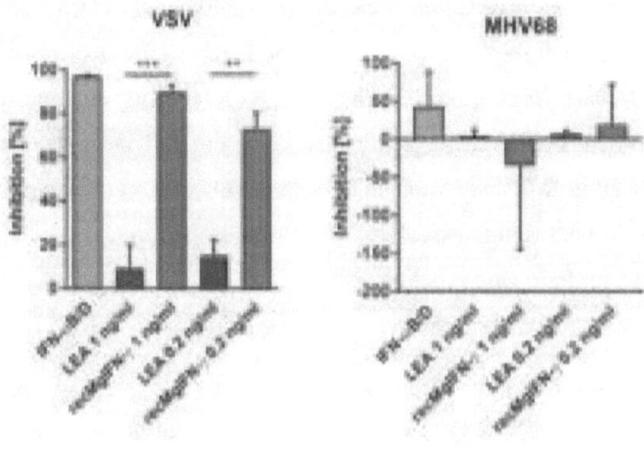

Fig. 25. rec*Mg*IFN-γ limits replication of vesicular stomatitis virus, but not of murine gammaherpesvirus 68, in BVK168 cells. Cells infected with either **(a)** VSV*ΔG(FLuc) or **(b)** MHV68 strains expressing firefly luciferase were treated with either IFN-αB/D (5 ng/ml) as a known positive effector; with two concentrations of rec*Mg*IFN-γ or the negative control protein LEA (1 and 0.2 ng/ml), or left untreated as control. The bioluminescence signal represents viral replication which is reported as percentage relative to untreated cells (not shown). Shown are mean ± SEM (n = 3 experiments, each with 2 or 3 replicates). Statistical analysis: One-way Anova (F(4, 10) = 37,24, p<0.0001) followed by Sidak's multiple comparisons test, ** p= 0.0003, *** p<0.0001.

6.2.6 Establishment of a bank vole reporter cell line responsive to rec*Mg*IFN-γ

An IFN-γ-responsive, sensitive reporter cell line would be advantageous for different purposes, like studying the influence of pathogens on JAK-STAT signalling pathway. Moreover, it would provide an easy system to test for functional activity of rec*Mg*IFN-γ. To this end, I established a bank vole reporter cell line from BVK168 cells (named BVK-LucA) containing the stably integrated pGAS-Luc-Bsd plasmid expressing firefly luciferase under the control of a minimal promoter with GAS sites (see chapter 5.4.2 for details on the establishment of the cell line). pGAS-Luc-Bsd encodes for a Renilla luciferase gene under the control of a promoter with a human-derived GAS sequence. The resulting plasmid pGAS-Luc-Bsd was transfected in BVK168 cells. Stimulation of BVK-LucA with an active IFN-γ induces expression of the luciferase via STAT1 binding to the GAS site. Thus, rec*Mg*IFN-γ activity can be tested on BVK-LucA cells in a bioluminescence assay.

Since this is the first stable transfection of bank vole cells to our knowledge, different transfection methods were tested. Methods included both polymer-based techniques, as home-produced polyethylenimine (PEI), and magnetic nanoparticles-conjugated reagents, as *PolyMag*™ and *CombiMag*™. All mentioned reagents are cationic polymers, or bound to cationic molecules, to bind the plasmid and introduce it in host cells (see 5.4.2 for details). BVK-LucA were transfected with the pmaxGFP plasmid to evaluate trasfection efficiency via expression of a green fluorescence protein. This bank vole cell line resulted easy to transfect with the highest efficiency reached with *PolyMag*™, followed by PEI and *CombiMag*™ (Fig. 26). Therefore, BVK168 cells were transfected with the created plasmid pGAS-Luc-Bsd independently with *PolyMag*™ and PEI methods, and selected for stable transfected clones. Cell growth and morphology were not affected, confirming *Magnetofection*™ and PEI-based methods suitable for transfection. The clonal BVK-LucA cell line established via PEI-transfection was used for following experiments.

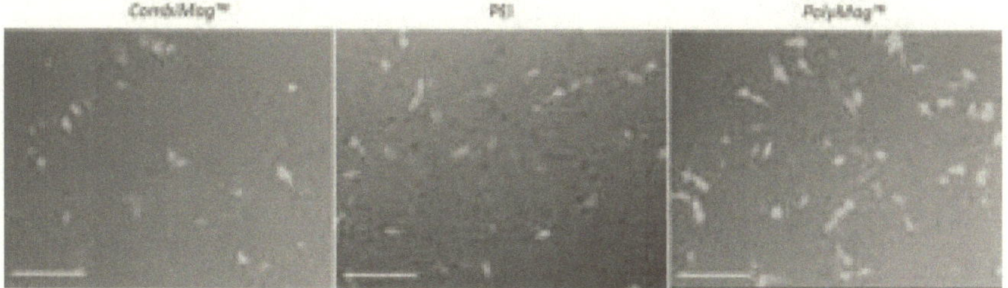

Fig. 26. Different transfection methods are suitable for the BVK168 bank vole cell line. BVK168 cells are easy to transfect and the Magnetofection™-based transfection method with *PolyMag*™ provides a higher transfection efficiency compared to *CombiMag*™ and polyethylenimine (PEI). BVK168 cells were transfected with the pmaxGFP plasmid expressing a green fluorescent cytoplasmic protein to evaluate transfection efficiency. Representative images are shown. The scale bar represents 200 μm.

The established BVK-LucA reporter cell line was treated with different concentrations of rec*Mg*IFN-γ in a bioluminescence assay to assess activity of the protein. Cells were treated with rec*Tg*LEA, mouse-γ and left untreated as control. As illustrated in Fig. 27a, titration of rec*Mg*IFN-γ produced a sigmoidal dose-response in bioluminescence (6 to 8-fold) relative to control cells, which is typical for bio-indicator lines. Within the linear range of the assay (between 20 and 0.02 ng/ml) rec*Mg*IFN-γ showed a dose-dependent decrease in signal strength, validating the BVK-LucA cell line as a useful tool to standardise rec*Mg*IFN-γ batches over a 100-fold concentration range.

After, I tested rec*Mg*IFN-γ activity from two independently produced batches of protein, each of them aliquoted in three different aliquots. Bioluminescence signal intensity resulting from the BVK-LucA treatment with all preparations was comparable 5 h post treatment, whereas up to 10-fold of difference in signal was observed at 18 h (Fig. 27b). Rec*Mg*IFN-γ aliquots giving comparable results at both time points, corresponding to n° 1 and 4 in Fig. 27b, were used all throughout the project.

I here for the first time established a stably transfected bank vole cell line. With the resulting BVK-LucA cells I confirmed the reproducibility in the activity of different batches of rec*Mg*IFN-γ. Treatment with the recombinant cytokine induces a dose-dependent bioluminescent signal in BVK-LucA cells, which could then be used to titrate the activity of different batches of protein.

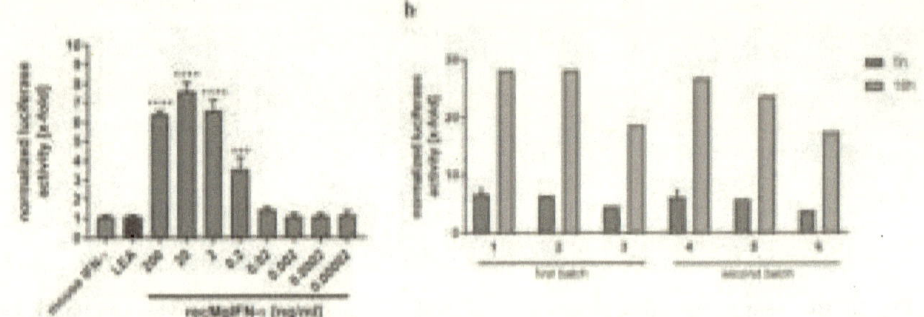

Fig. 27. Dose-dependent firefly luciferase activity after recMgIFN-γ induction in a bank vole reporter cell line. Bioluminescence assay on the reporter cell line BVK-LucA expressing the firefly luciferase gene under the control of a GAS promoter element. The reported bioluminescence values are relative to untreated cells. **(a)** Cells were either left untreated (ctrl, not shown) or treated with the control protein LEA (200 ng/ml); mouse IFN-γ (200 ng/ml) or recMgIFN-γ (200 to 0.00002 ng/ml). Mean ± SEM (n = 4 experiments, each with 3 replicates). Statistical analysis: One-way Anova (F(9, 30) = 76,16, p= <0.0001) followed by Dunnett's multiple comparisons test (all against the LEA control protein). *** p=0.0002, **** p≤0.0001, relative to the control protein LEA. Note that only statistically significant (p≤0.05) differences were depicted in the figure. **(b)** Rec*Mg*IFN-γ activity in different produced batches is comparable. Cells were either left untreated (ctrl, not shown) or treated for 5 h and 18 h with two different batches of rec*Mg*IFN-γ (200 ng/ml), each aliquoted in three different vessels. Variance indicates ± sd of 2 independent experiments.

6.3　*T. gondii* infection in *M. glareolus*-derived cell cultures

6.3.1　Virulent *T. gondii* growth in the BVK168 bank vole cell line

The number of established non-model cell lines is constantly increasing (57); however is still very limited compared to classical hosts like human and *Mus* spp.. Thus, the availability of an established *M. glareolus* kidney cell line (BVK168, (125)) represented a fortunate starting point to study parasite growth in this rodent species. Susceptibility to different virus infections has been already established in this cell line (125); however to our knowledge the work presented here is the first parasite infection performed in bank vole cells.

To test the hypothesis that vole cells resist virulent T. gondii infection via an IFN-γ-dependent mechanism, we first observed parasite virulence in BVK168 cells in a so-called plaque assay. Parasite growth is assessed by quantifying the number of infection foci, or plaques. A host-induced limitation of parasite growth results in less such plaques (Fig. 28a). Surprisingly, BVK168 cells treated with rec*Mg*IFN-γ had an identical number of plaques to untreated controls, but of larger size (Fig. 28b). A direct comparison with murine fibroblasts was not possible since the latter outgrown the formed plaques (not shown), contrary to vole kidney cells which grow as a monolayer. Since BVK168 cells do not reach full confluence, but rather leave small openings, the assay was only performed with RHβGFPmt parasite strain which expresses β-galactosidase and allows a distinction between spontaneous cavities and *T. gondii* induced plaques (see Fig 28a).

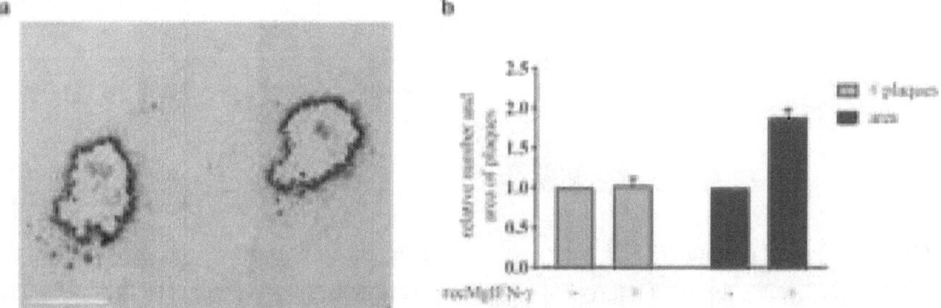

Fig. 28. Virulent *T. gondii* infection leads to bigger plaques in rec*Mg*IFN-γ-treated BVK168 cells. *M. glareolus* BVK168 cells were treated with 200 ng/ml rec*Mg*IFN-γ or left untreated 24 h prior infection with type I *T. gondii* strain expressing β-galactosidase for plaque assay. **(a)** Vole BVK168 cells are suitable for plaque assay since cells grow as monolayer. Parasites were stained with X-Gal/NBT staining (179). The scale bar represents 500 μm. **(b)** Mean ± sd of plaque number and area, normalized to untreated controls (n = 2 experiments, each with 2 or 3 replicates).

6.3.2 *T. gondii* inhibits STAT1 pathway in bank vole cells

Recently it was unveiled that *T. gondii* manipulation of the host acts also via inhibition of the IFN-γ pathway by blocking STAT1 transcriptional activity, observed in both human and murine cells. *T. gondii* TgIST sequesters STAT1 in an inactive form within the host nucleus, blocking its transcriptional activity (88, 89). The availability of the bank vole reporter cell line BVK-LucA allowed us to test whether the parasite's ability is exclusive for mouse and human cells, or whether it is a conserved feature also in other rodents such as *M. glareolus*. With this assay, cells exhibit bioluminescence upon IFN-γ treatment due to STAT1 binding to the GAS sequences in the promoter region of the luciferase gene. Cells were infected prior to IFN-γ treatment similarly to published protocols (88). Parasite infection of both virulent and avirulent strains decreased the bioluminescence signal induced by rec*Mg*IFN-γ, indicating that parasites inhibit the STAT1 pathway similarly to previous reports on *Mus* species (Fig. 29).

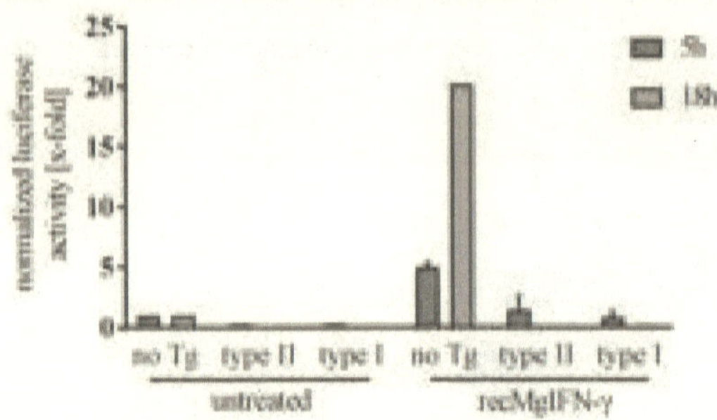

Fig. 29. *T. gondii* inhibits STAT1 pathway in vole cells. Bioluminescence assay on the reporter cell line BVK-LucA at 5 h and 18 h post-treatment. Cells were either infected with type I (RhßGFPmt) or type II (Pru dtTomato) *T. gondii* strains or left uninfected. 2 h post infection, cells were either treated with rec*Mg*IFN-γ (400 ng/ml) or left untreated. The reported bioluminescence values are relative to untreated not infected cells. Variance indicates ± sd of 2 independent experiments, each with 3 technical replicates.

6.3.3   Establishment of primary *M. glareolus* cell culture systems

Although another kidney cell line is commonly used for *T. gondii* infection – i.e. the African green monkey VERO cell line – kidney cells are not likely to play a major role in vivo. The most used cell types for *in vitro* tachyzoite infection are immune cells such as macrophages (180) and nonhemopoietic cells as fibroblasts. Both hemopoietic and non hemopoietic cells are crucial for cellular immune response to *T. gondii* infection (74). The fortunate access in my institute to a living colony of *M. glareolus* gave us the chance to expand the repertoire of available relevant cell types. Notably, this is the first reported attempt of isolation of *M. glareolus* immune cells.

Protocols for establishment of *M. glareolus* Bone Marrow-Derived Macrophages (BMDMs) and primary fibroblasts systems (explained in Chapter 5.3.2) required several steps of optimization. Final protocols reported here lead to BMDM cultures which phenotypically resemble murine BMDMs. To evaluate their phenotype, BMDMs were incubated with latex beads to test for phagocytic activity (181). I observed equal distribution of macrophages in four different categories according to their phagocytic capacity: a quarter had the cytoplasm full of beads, a quarter counted between three and ten beads, a quarter had only one or two beads per cell and the remaining quarter phagocytized no beads at all (Fig. 30a). Additionally, phenotypic characterization of BMDMs by flow cytometry was attempted using antibodies against specific markers, e.g. CD68 and F4/80, but was unsuccessful (data not shown).

As anticipated from results on BVK168 cells, both cell cultures were responsive to rec*Mg*IFN-γ, as indicated by the phosphorylation of the nuclear STAT1 in treated cells compared to untreated controls (Fig 30b, controls not shown).

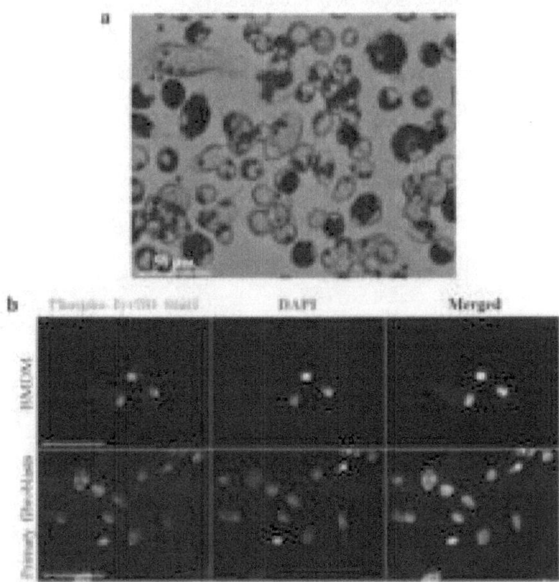

Fig. 30. *M. glareolus* **Bone Marrow-Derived Macrophages (BMDMs) and primary fibroblasts cultures were established. (a)** Phagocytic assay with BMDMs and latex beads. A representative image is shown. **(b)** Both cultures are responsive to rec*Mg*IFN-γ as indicated by phosphorylation and translocation to the nucleus of STAT1 following treatment (200 ng/ml) compared to untreated controls (not shown). In each panel, the following stainings are shown from left to right: phospho-Tyr701-STAT1 staining (green), DAPI staining for nuclei (white) and overlay of the two signals. A representative experiment of three replicates is shown. The scale bar represents 50 μm.

6.3.4 Virulent *T. gondii* growth in *M. glareolus* cell cultures

T. gondii replicates synchronously in a binary logarithmic fashion, resulting in vacuoles with a single, two, four, or eight or more parasites, until they egress from the infected cell. First evidence of host resistance is represented by a decrease in the number of parasites per vacuole following immune activation (182). To test the hypothesis that primary and immortalized vole cells resist virulent parasites infection in an IFN-γ-dependent manner we monitored intracellular parasite growth at two times points post infection: at 24 h and 36 h, with and without treatment with rec*Mg*IFN-γ.

Rec*Mg*IFN-γ treatment does not seem to impact parasite replication at 24 hpi in BMDMs and BVK168 cells, but it results in bigger vacuoles in BMDM at 36 hpi (Fig. 31a and 31b). On the contrary, preliminary results on primary fibroblasts display the opposite trend, with parasites replicating faster following rec*Mg*IFN-γ treatment compared to untreated controls at 24 hpi. However, this difference in numbers is not observable twelve hours later (Fig. 31c). Notably, the majority of vacuoles with eight parasites or more observed in BMDM cultures were in big polynucleated cells (black arrow head in Fig. 31d), whereas most of the smaller cells with a single nucleus had one parasite or none. These polynucleated cells, or giant cells, increased in number upon infection, suggesting an induction following infection. Taken together, in the *M. glareolus* host parasite intracellular growth is not strongly influenced by rec*Mg*IFN-γ treatment in any of the cell types investigated here, in spite of STAT1 activation.

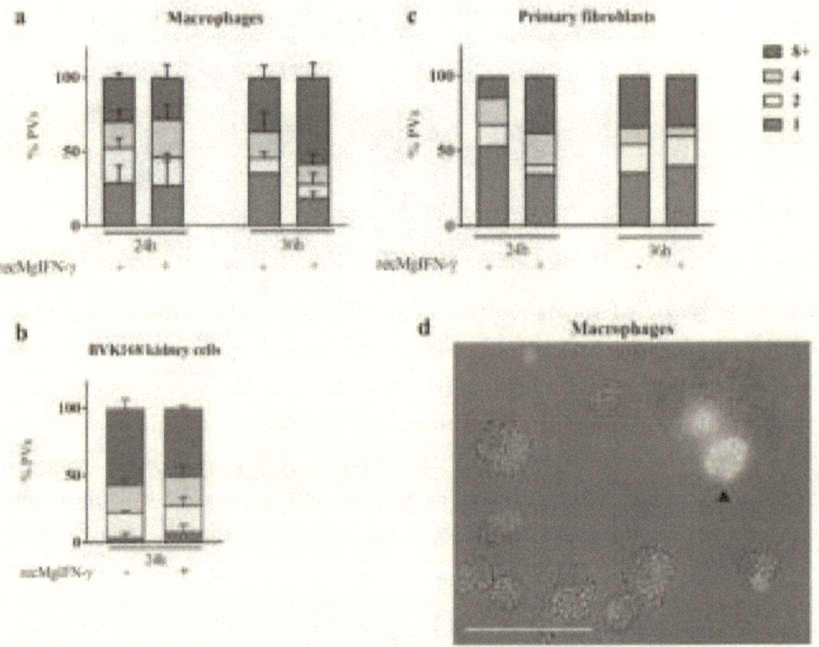

Fig. 31. Virulent parasite intracellular growth is not decreased in *M. glareolus* cells following rec*Mg*IFN-γ treatment. I investigated three different *M. glareolus* cell cultures: **(a)** Bone Marrow-Derived Macrophages (BMDMs), **(b)** an immortalized BVK168 kidney cell line, and **(c)** primary fibroblasts. Cells were treated with 200 ng/ml rec*Mg*IFN-γ or left untreated 24 h prior to infection with type I *T. gondii* expressing a green fluorescent protein in the mitochondria. 24 hpi and 36 hpi cells were fixed, parasites' plasma membrane stained to facilitate counting parasites per vacuole. The number of parasites was counted in at least 100 parasitophorous vacuoles per sample. Mean ± sd (n = 2 experiments) is shown. **(d)** shows a representative immunofluorescent assay of recMgIFN-γ-treated

BMDM 36 hpi. The black arrow-head indicates the vacuole containing more than eight parasites in a multinucleated cell. A Differential Interference Contrast (DIC) transmission light image with overlay of the following stainings is shown: parasite mitochondria marker (green), parasite membrane with anti-SAG1 staining (red) and DAPI staining of nuclei (blue). The scale bar represents 50 μm.

6.3.5   IFN-γ-mediated cell death during *T. gondii* infection

Host-mediated parasite killing followed by death of the host cell itself was proposed as a host resistance mechanism. Because BVK168 cells infected with virulent parasites were observed rounding up and detaching from the plate bottom in rec*Mg*IFN-γ-treated but not in untreated control cells (not shown), I hypothesized that this phenomenon occurs in vole cells as well. I measured the magnitude of host cell death in several cell types during infection by means of two assays as described below.

Propidium Iodide assay to detect host cell death during *T. gondii* infection

We performed a double staining with Propidium Iodide (PI) and Hoechst 33342 to quantify the ratio of necrotic (PI+) cells during *T. gondii* infection and IFN-γ stimulation. All *M. glareolus* cells displayed an IFN-γ-dependant increase in cell death during virulent infection (Fig. 32 a and b). This phenotype is therefore conserved in all these species cells; however, to different degrees depending on cell type. Almost all type I infected primary fibroblasts died, more than half of BMDM cells died, and ~20 % kidney cells of the immortalized BVK168 cell line died as determined by the PI-assay. During avirulent infection only primary fibroblasts showed an increase in cell death in IFN-γ-treated cells compared to untreated controls.

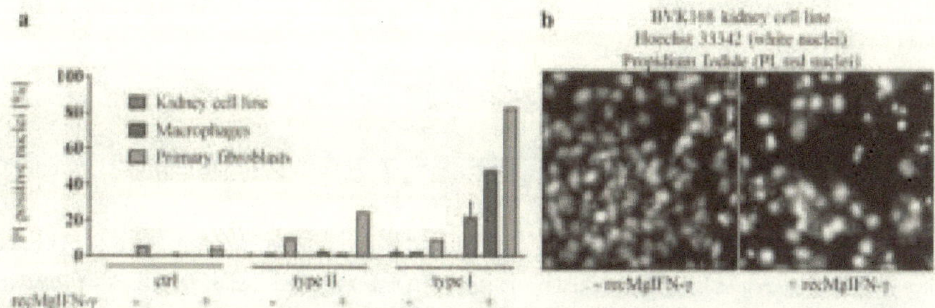

Fig. 32. *M. glareolus* cells undergo IFN-γ-mediated cell death following virulent *T. gondii*-infection. (a) *M. glareolus* BVK168 kidney cell line, Bone Marrow-Derived Macrophages (BMDMs), and primary fibroblasts were treated with 200 ng/ml rec*Mg*IFN-γ or left untreated 24 h prior infection with avirulent (type II) and virulent (type I) *T. gondii*. 24 hpi a double staining with Propidium Iodide (PI) and Hoechst 33342 on living cells was performed and double stained nuclei were quantified at the fluorescent microscope. Variance indicate mean ± sd (n = 3 experiments, each with 2 technical replicates). **(b)** Representative image of BVK168 cells infected with RhßmGFP type I parasites expressing a green fluorescent protein in the mitochondria.

Flow cytometry-based assay to detect host cell death and *T. gondii* parasite burden

The performed experiments informed us that IFN-γ-primed *M. glareolus* cells die following virulent parasite infection while the intracellular growth in surviving cells seems not to be affected. However, we did not have information regarding the overall *T. gondii* burden changes following treatment. We decided to develop an appropriate assay to assess this and further prove the IFN-γ-related cell death. A LIVE/DEAD fixable dye, staining exclusively dying cells, was used in a flow cytometry-based experiment as described in chapter 5.3.7 and showed in Fig. 33a. Infection with differently fluorescent parasite strains allowed their detection with appropriate lasers, whereas the cell population was recognized by its physical parameters.

The performed experiments informed us that IFN-γ-primed *M. glareolus* cells die following virulent parasite infection whereas the intracellular growth in surviving cells does not seem to be affected. However, the PI-assay does not assess the overall *T. gondii* burden changes following treatment. I developed an assay to assess this and further investigate IFN-γ-related host cell death. A LIVE/DEAD fixable dye, staining exclusively dying cells, was used in a flow cytometry-based experiment as described in chapter 5.3.7 and shown in Fig. 33a. Infection with differently fluorescent parasite strains allowed detection with appropriate lasers, whereas the host cell population was recognized by its physical parameters.

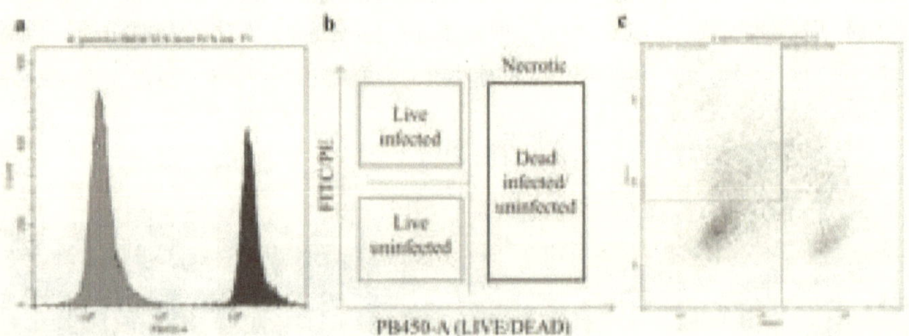

Fig. 33. Gating strategy for the flow cytometry-based assay. (a) A mixed population of living and heat-killed *M. glareolus* BMDMs stained with the LIVE/DEAD dye detected by the PB450-A filter. **(b)** Gating strategy of live infected, live uninfected and necrotic cells, the latter including both infected and uninfected populations. On the y axis either the FITC or the PE channel, according to the infection performed with either RHβGFPmt (type I) or Pru tdTomato (type II) parasites respectively. **(c)** An example of gating on rec*Mg*IFN-γ-treated *M. glareolus* BMDM 8 hpi with RHβGFPmt.

The assay was performed in *M. glareolus* BMDMs since they displayed a more pronounced phenotype than kidney cells in the PI-assay and posed less challenges in cultures compared to primary fibroblasts. Confirming the PI-assay results, an IFN-γ-dependent increase in dying BMDMs of 50 % compared to untreated controls was observed during virulent parasite infection (Fig. 34a). At the same time, the amount of living infected cells, which would further contribute to infection in a real setting, decreased drastically. Also, confirming the phenotype with avirulent parasite infection, an increase in cell death was not measured with type II parasite infection. However, IFN-γ-treated cells appear able to clear infection since the amount of infected cells was halved 24 hpi (Fig. 34a). In living infected cells the median fluorescence intensity relative to the parasite labels for type I and type II parasites, decreased by almost 40 % compared to untreated cells (Fig. 34b). The same trend was visible already at 8 hpi in two independently performed experiments (Fig. 34c). Taken together these results indicate that *M. glareolus* BMDM limit both virulent and avirulent parasites burden in a IFN-γ-dependent fashion.

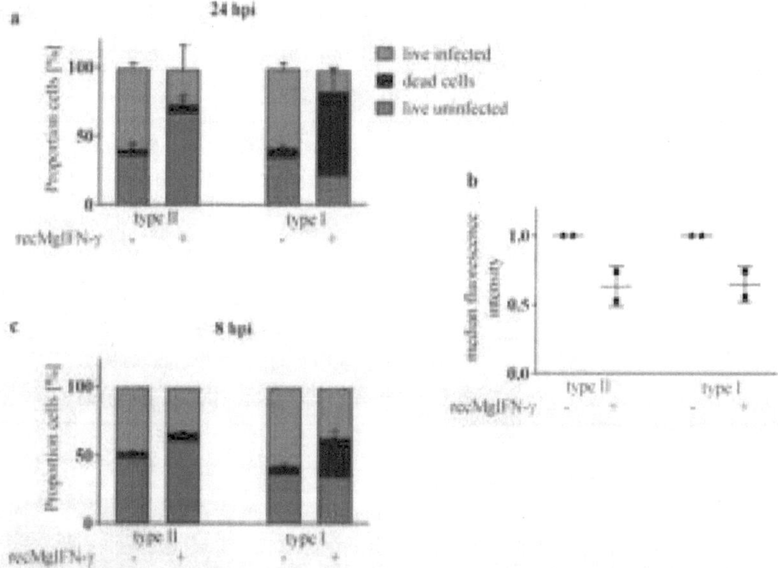

Fig. 34. IFN-γ treatment decreases parasite burden in *M. glareolus* Bone Marrow-Derived Macrophages. *M. glareolus* Bone Marrow-Derived Macrophages were treated with 200 ng/ml recMgIFN-γ or left untreated 24 h prior infection with type II and type I *T. gondii* strains. **(a)** 24 hpi cells were stained with a LIVE/DEAD dye, fixed and analyzed at the flow-cytometer. Mean ± sd (n = 2 experiments, each with 2 replicates). **(b)** Decrease in the median fluorescence of live infected cells in recMgIFN-γ-treated cells indicates a decrease in parasite burden. **(c)** Same experiment performed at 8 hpi. Mean ± sd (n = 2 experiments, each with 2 replicates).

6.3.6 Investigating the role of *M. glareolus* Immunity Related GTPases in resistance to *T. gondii*

Results support *M. glareolus* resistance to both virulent and avirulent *T. gondii* infection in a IFN-γ-dependant fashion. This phenotype is related to IFN-γ-induced mediators. Since our main protein family of interest, IRG, is induced by the cytokine, we investigated the possible role of IRGs as mediators. Unfortunately, antibodies developed against the murine proteins do not cross-react with this vole species (Tab. 19), making it impossible to directly study IRGs in *M. glareolus*-derived cells without developing species-specific antibodies. As for the main target, IRGb2-b1, a small band is visible in a Western Blot with lysates from IFN-γ treated BVK168 cells. However, this faint band is not comparable with the one visible for the positive control murine cells, and could even be another recognized tandem, similarly to what I observed in Flp Δb2b1 in Fig. 18a.

Tab. 19 List of murine antibodies and serum anti-murine Irg proteins tested on *M. musculus* and *M. glareolus* cell lines. The type of parasite used during infection in IFA, either I or II, is reported in parenthesis. When not specified, the experiment performed was an IFA. * This experiment was performed by Tobias Steinfeldt (183). Na = not assessed. Detailes on antibodies sources are indicated in Tab. 6. [§] indicates the commercial anti-IRGb6 antibody.

Species	Cell lines	IRGa6	IRGb6	IRGb6 [§]	IRGb2-b1	IRGb10*
M. musculus	NIH/3T3 and Flp-In-3T3	✓ (II) Fig. 35b	✓ (II)	✓ (I and II)	✗ (I and II) IFA ✓ WB	na
M. glareolus	BVK168 and BMDM	✗ (II)	✗ (II)	✗ (I and II)	✗ (I and II) not clear WB, Fig. 35a	✓ WB

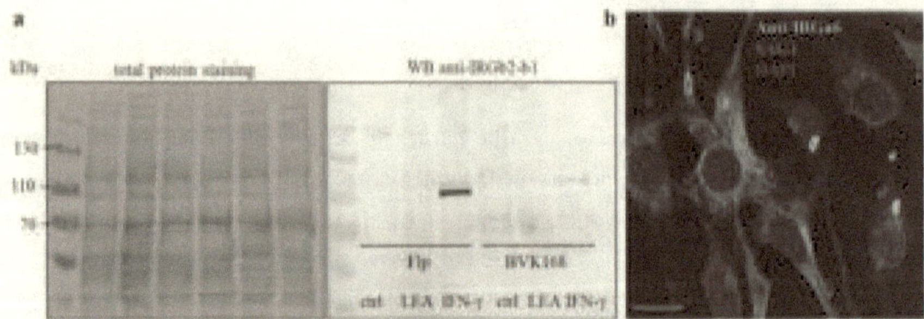

Fig. 35. There is no cross-reactivity of murine anti-IRG antibodies with vole cell lines. (a) DB71 total protein staining (left) and Western Blot with anti-IRGb2-b1 serum on the same membrane (right) of lysates from Flp-In-3T3 and BVK168 cells. Cells were treated for 24 h with IFN-γ (mouse IFN-γ 200 U/ml for Flp-In-3T3 cells and rec*Mg*IFN-γ 200 ng/ml for BVK168 cells), with the negative control protein rec*Tg*LEA (LEA, 200 ng/ml) or left untreated as control (ctrl). The first lane is the molecular weight marker (with sizes in kDa given to the left). **(b)** IFA of NIH/3T3 cells infected with type II *T.*

gondii. The following stainings are shown: *T. gondii* SAG1 (red), GRA7 (green), DAPI staining for nuclei (blue). A representative image is shown. The scale bar represents 20 µm.

Therefore, to study the role IRGs play for the *M. glareolus* resistance phenotype, I first applied the cell culture-based system developed in this book and presented in chapter 6.1.5. However, as already shown, we were not able to replicate results from literature with regards to positive and negative control cell lines. Therefore, we did not pursue the use of the cell culture system in this context.

We overcame this problem by using another recently published cell-based system (115). Using CRISPR-Cas9, the group of Tobias Steinfeldt (University of Freiburg, Germany) established a clonal CIM Δb2b1 cell line lacking *Irgb2-b1*$_{CIM,}$ which renders the cells susceptible to virulent parasite infection. The cell line is a useful tool to screen resistant *Irg* genes, since reintroduction of *Irgb2-b1*$_{CIM}$ rescues host resistance to virulent parasites. We decided to complement CIM Δb2b1 with the cloned vole tandem *Irgb2-b1* from BVK168 cells, herein named *Irgb2-b1*$_{BVK}$ (see sequence in Fig. 9). This allows me to assess the vole IRGb2-b1 phenotype during infection in otherwise susceptible cells. Preliminary analysis of the RNAseq data of BVK168 IFN-γ-induced cells (chapter 6.1.3) identified the cloned *Irgb2-b1*$_{BVK}$ gene in the transcripts. The identified wild type gene has three different amino acids caused by SNPs in the primer binding regions which were corrected before cloning. Furthermore, the last three codons missing at the C-terminal because of the SapI site (as explained in chapter 6.1.5.1) were introduced. Two different clonal cell lines were established: the first with the *Irgb2-b1*$_{BVK}$ wild type sequence (CIM Δb2b1-*Irgb2-b1*$_{BVK}$) and the second with the same in frame with an HA-tag (CIM Δb2b1-*Irgb2-b1*$_{BVK}$ HA). Gene insertion was performed by Steinfeldt according to published protocols (115). As visible in Fig. 36, the established CIM Δb2b1-*Irgb2-b1*$_{BVK}$ HA cell line constitutively expresses an HA-tag protein at the size of IRGb2-b1, confirming successful cloning of the gene. Confirming our results in Fig. 35a, the anti-IRGb2-b1 antibody does not cross-react with the vole tandem IRG-like protein in CIM Δb2b1-*Irgb2-b1*$_{BVK}$ cells (Fig. 36). Experiments on the resistance phenotype associated with the introduced gene are currently being performed and evaluated.

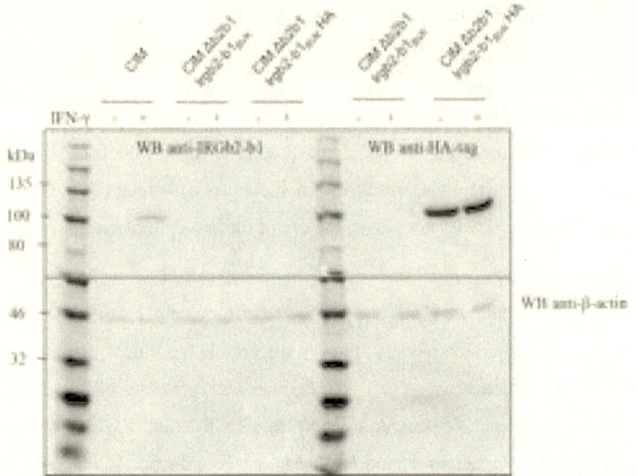

Fig. 36. Creation of clonal cell lines expressing vole IRGb2-b1. Western Blot with anti-tandem IRG serum, anti-HA-tag and anti-β-actin of lysates from CIM, CIM Δb2b1-Irgb2-b1$_{BVK}$ and CIM Δb2b1-Irgb2-b1$_{BVK}$ HA cells. Cells were treated for 24 h with mouse IFN-γ 200 U/ml or left untreated as control. First and eight lanes with molecular weight marker (with sizes in kDa given to the left). The Western Blot was performed by Tobias Steinfeldt (University of Freiburg, Germany).

7. Discussion

Wildlife has a recognized central role in zoonotic transmissions (184) of which small mammals alone are responsible of nearly 60 % (185). Within Rodentia, voles are a reservoir for 20 % of zoonotic pathogens and are predicted to gain even more relevance in the near future (186). Whereas research on zoonotic potentials in the fields of viruses and bacteria is proceeding, identification of eukaryotic parasitic reservoirs in nature is still neglected (184). In the last two decades, a considerably small number of works focused on *T. gondii* prevalence in Mammals have been published (187). Therefore, research on parasitic infections in small mammals, particularly in voles, requires further investigation. This book makes a contribution to this field by investigating the potential of wild rodents, in particular voles as *M. glareolus* and *Microtus* spp., as reservoirs for *T. gondii* in Europe.

Further adding to their research value as natural reservoirs for pathogens, voles are gaining interest in the expanding field of wild or eco-immunology. This branch of immunology focuses on gaining new insights on immunologic systems by mimicking natural contexts (57). The add-on derives from either the direct study of natural populations or by using wild-derived systems in experiments performed in a controlled environment. The vast majority of research studies in biology, including infection biology, are based on the use of *M. musculus* as model organism. Despite the crucial role of laboratory mouse systems for advancing in basic biological knowledge, an increasing body of evidence highlights the numerous inadequacies of this model (as described for example in these studies (57, 188, 189)). A published review which I co-authored (58) and in which we collected results from numerous studies, reports issues encountered when using *M. musculus* as a model for biomedical research, arguing for caution in the use of this and other animal models. In the specific example of *T. gondii* research, the definition of parasite virulence in laboratory mice does not reflect the natural susceptibility of *M. musculus* to *T. gondii* infection. Lilue et al. showed that the extensive inbreeding of *T. gondii* mouse models led to the genomic conservation of *Irg* genotypes which are associated with a susceptible phenotype to infection. This does not reflect the high natural variability of *Irg* genes which is comparable to that of the Major Histocompatibility Complex (MHC, (7)). The study of Lilue et al. evidences how the use of laboratory models influenced conclusions on mouse susceptibility in nature, which should be revised. In Ehret et al. we also suggest alternatives to the use of laboratory inbred strains. Rodents of *M. glareolus*, *Microtus* spp. and *Apodemus* spp. have already been suggested as possible models for infection studies. These rodent species are largely diffused, they are natural reservoirs of numerous zoonotic pathogens, and carry the genetic variability lacking in inbred mice (51, 188, 189). Both wild rodents and wild-derived colonies can help identifying genes linked to susceptibility to pathogens (190). The main drawback with using non-model organisms is the lack of genomic references and tested reagents, opposite to the murine model that has a long-established set of tools. Nevertheless, significant technological advancements combined with an increasing attention from the scientific community are helping filling this gap (57, 189). Here, we provide new tools, namely the recombinant vole IFN-γ and a reporter cell line to assess its activity, as well as novel cell culture-based systems, to foster research on non-model species. I also want to emphasize the need for similar models particularly in the field of parasitology, which is concerned with pathogens with commonly complex life cycles and which per definition infect several hosts.

In the context of research on *T. gondii*, it has already been suggested that wildlife, particularly rodent species different from *M. musculus*, might be important reservoir for persistence of certain genotypes (191). Indeed, in a recent study Galal et al. show that autochthonous non-murine rodent species in Senegal are tolerant to infection with virulent *T. gondii* genotypes, and develop chronic infection (192). On the contrary, the same parasite genotypes do not infect *M. musculus* despite sampling in the same geographical area. The authors speculate that the more recent arrival of *M. musculus*, imported during the Colonial era, did not allow for co-evolution processes between host and pathogen. This work highlights the need to foster research in natural, non-laboratory systems. The same co-evolution mechanism was suggested for virulent *T. gondii*, such as RH and GT1 strains, and wild-derived *M. musculus castaneus* from Asia, where these genotypes are more common (7). Interestingly, Hassan et al. recently showed that the locus encompassing the *Irg* genes was associated with resistance not only in *M. musculus castaneus* species, but also in the other subspecies *M. musculus musculus*, regardless of breeding approach (62). On the contrary, *M. musculus domesticus*, whose genome is conserved in 92 % (including loci for *Irgs*) of laboratory inbred strains (193), displays susceptibility to virulent infection. This work further highlights the critical protective role of IRG proteins during *T. gondii* infection in a relevant host such as *M. musculus*.

With the current work we provided new tools to approach research on the non-model organism *M. glareolus* and closely related voles. Furthermore, we investigated the role of non-murine rodent species as intermediate hosts for virulent *T. gondii* genotypes in Europe. We considered *M. glareolus*, *Microtus* spp. and *Apodemus* spp. since they are major prey of the domestic cat. Moreover, current data indicate that these three rodent groups display lower susceptibility to and higher prevalence of *T. gondii* compared to the more often studied *Mus* spp. Considering the major role of the IRG immune response in mediating resistance in certain *M. musculus* subspecies, we hypothesized that the same mechanism is conserved in these other rodents species.

7.1 Development of a cell culture-based system to study *Irg*-like genes in non-murine wild rodents

7.1.1 *Irg*-like genes variability in wild rodents

The complexity of *Irg* sequences, together with the lack of good genomic references, constituted a real challenge to obtain an overview of this gene family in non-murine rodents. The RNAseq data currently in analysis will provide a comprehensive picture of expressed *Irg*-like genes in the available wild rodents-derived cell lines. In the recent years transcriptomic analysis made remarkable advances and data annotation of non-model organisms is now approachable (189). Transcriptomic data will allow us to design specific primers to amplify individual *Irg*-like genes. The highly repetitive nature of *Irg* genes poses an extra challenge: it is not possible to us to discriminate between different alleles of the same gene or two similar genes in two distinct loci, for which availability of a relative genome is necessary. For this reason, I couldn't draw conclusions about the correspondence between cloned tandem *Irg*-like genes from cDNA and identical sequences from cloned gDNA, as in the case of AAL-R tandem 1 (Fig. 8a), since gene duplication cannot be excluded. A good annotated genome is likely to be provided for bank voles in the near future, given the common interest of other groups (Rainer Ulrich, personal communication). In this project I cloned and sequenced single *Irg*-like genes, which is a tedious and time-consuming approach. Furthermore, PCR amplification of *Irg*-like sequences from gut-derived gDNA was largely unsuccessful (Fig. 10b). Many reasons could account for the lack of PCR products: lack of binding of the primers, presence of an excessive amount of inhibitors as already observed for *CytB* amplification (Fig. 10a), or amplification below detection limit since the genes are single-copy. Availability of gDNA derived from tissues other than the intestine with less PCR inhibitors would be beneficial for the project. I suggest for future work to streamline the collection of *Irg*-like sequences via for example meta-barcoding, which allows pooling of different samples and is possible for non-model organisms, as recently reviewed by Schoetterer et al. (194). For example, the T cell receptor (TCR) variability was characterized via high-throughput sequencing in a collection of *M. glareolus* samples (195). Profiling of immune genes, like *TCR*, *Irg* and *MHC*, will surely foster immunological studies in relevant reservoirs in the wild. Successful examples are given by studies reporting a correlation between specific *MHC* alleles and nematode infection in *M. glareolus* (196) and genetic diversity of different cytokines and infection with several pathogens in a well-studied population of *M. agrestis* (121). Different polymorphisms and expression levels of host immune genes might ultimately lead to differences in the geographic distribution of pathogens (119). I envisage that, with this established set-up, we will be able to identify immune genes correlated with infection to *T. gondii* in German samples of *M. glareolus*, *Microtus* spp. and *Apodemus* spp. already available to us (49).

Despite resource limitation, I increased knowledge about putative *Irg* genes in non-murine rodents. First, analysis of the *M. ochrogaster* transcriptome revealed that *Irg*-like genes disposition is conserved with *Mus musculus* (Fig. 6). Putative effector genes and two tandem *Irg*-like genes are present in this vole species. Their presence hints to a possible role in cell-autonomous defense against intracellular pathogens like *T. gondii*, since not relevant intermediate hosts like humans lost the genes (197). Tandem *Irg*-like genes are not only expressed in *M. ochrogaster*, but also in our German wild rodents-derived cell lines (Fig. 7). Several results indicate the presence of more than one putative tandem-*Irg* in these rodent species: *Irg*-like genomic loci are amplified as 9 and 11 kb-long PCR products and are transcribed as 2.5 kb-long mRNA (Fig. 8a and 8b). The two bands from PCR-amplied gDNA were observed for murine Flp-In-3T3 cells, *M. arvalis* FMN-R cells and *A. agrarius* AAL-R cells, and have a similar size to those of reference *M. musculus* and *M. ochrogaster* genomes. In spite of the presence of a single band for *M. glareolus* BVK168 cells, we cannot exclude presence of more than one tandem since introns might vary in size. Furthermore, *Irg*-genes heterozygosity was observed in wild-derived *M. musculus* ((163), Jonathan Howard personal communication) and could characterize our samples as well. Mixed nucleotides from sequencing of PCR products for all the mentioned wild rodent species confirm the presence of more than one putative tandem *Irg* gene or allele (Fig. 8c). The *A. agrarius* tandem 2 IRG-like protein is characterized by many stop codons at the C-terminal (Fig. 9). Further work will assess whether the repetitive residues in the sequence caused a frame-shift (Appendix Fig. 37) or if the gene is a pseudogene, whose presence in the *Irg* family has already been described in *Mus* spp. (7). Future availability of good quality genomic and transcriptomic data of the same cell lines will help to interprete these results.

I observed that the IRGb2-like subunit only (with the C-terminal of IRGb1) binds the PVM of virulent parasites (Fig. 15b). This observation recalls published results from Murillo-Leon et al. on the IRGb2$_{CIM}$-subunit, which is sufficient for binding and to confer resistance in *in vitro* infections (115). They concluded that the molecular mechanism of resistance resides within residues in the *Irgb2* exon. We observed variability in the IRGb2-like subunit of wild rodents' samples, in residues where the resistant IRGb2$_{CIM}$ differs from the susceptible IRGb2$_{BL6}$ (Fig. 11). Notably, these different residues are enriched at the putative interface with *T. gondii* virulence factor ROP5, suggesting positive selection at this site (Fig. 12). The highest amino acid diversity between IRGb2$_{CIM}$ and IRGb2$_{BL6}$ was observed in the αD and H4 domains (7), which are also diverse in our wild rodents' samples (Fig. 9). Analysis of a higher number of samples is necessary to support the hypothesis of positive selection in these domains and to identify putative critical residues for resistance.

Polymorphisms directly influencing host susceptibility to infection can also be found in genes upstream in the pathway leading to *Irg* genes expression. For example Rohfritsch et al. found polymorphisms in TLR and JAK-STAT-associated genes, e.g. IL12rb1, in a wild population of *M. glareolus* to be associated with tolerance to Puumala virus infection (198). Similar mechanisms might exist for infection with other pathogens, as the protozoan *T. gondii*. Also SNPs in non-coding regions could affect gene expression and lead to different susceptibility to infection. *M. glareolus* SNPs in non-coding regions of the immune related gene IFIH1, important for virus sensing, influence its expression levels (199).

7.1.2   Not reproducibility of the resistance phenotype in the positive control cell line

I developed the Flp-In-3T3-based cell system to investigate the phenotype related to IRG-like proteins from wild rodents during infection with *T. gondii*. I first tested the system by establishing a positive control cell line expressing the resistant *Irgb2-b1*$_{CIM}$ and a negative control cell line expressing the susceptible *Irgb2-b1*$_{BL6}$ (Fig. 14a). I expected the created Flp-CIM and Flp-BL6 to be resistant and susceptible to virulent T. gondii infection respectively. In Table 20 I graphically summarize the outcome of *in vitro* infections performed on murine and vole cell systems in this project. I compare my results to published work on inbred mouse cells and wild-derived *M. musculus castaneus* cells. In literature, IFN-γ-treated BL6 murine embryonic fibroblasts (MEFs) drastically decrease type II *T. gondii* parasite burden and display an increase of 25 % in necrotic cells compared to untreated control cells at 24 hpi (7). This *in vitro* phenotype is correlated with host resistance *in vivo* and we refer to it as the "resistance phenotype" (7). *M. musculus castaneus* CIM strain display the same *in vitro* phenotype to infection with both medium virulent type II and virulent type I strains, and are resistant to the same *in vivo* (7, 115). Therefore, data from literature suggest that host resistance is linked to IFN-γ-mediated host cell death. On the contrary, BL6 MEFs limit parasite burden of type I *T. gondii* but do not undergo cell death (7).

Since infection with the same strain *in vivo* is lethal for inbred mice, we refer to the lack of host cell death as the "susceptible phenotype".

Tab. 20. Infection phenotype with virulent and intermediate virulent *T. gondii* in vole and murine systems. A graphical report of the performed *in vitro* experiments in this study and published work on inbred mouse cells and wild-derived *M. musculus castaneus* cells. Highlighted in pink the cell types that display >20 % cell death to type I T. gondii infection. This *in vitro* phenotype is associated in *M. musculus castaneus* CIM mice with *in vivo* resistance to type I infection. Reported *in vitro* assays are diverse. Host cell death expressed in percentage was detected by Propidium Iodide staining in this study, whereas in published work was deducted from cell viability assays. *T. gondii* burden was quantified in a flow-cytometry-based assay in this as well as published work; other works also quantified parasite burden by ^{3}H-uracil incorporation or *T. gondii*-mediated enzymatic reactions. *T. gondii* intracellular (IC) growth refers to the number of parasites counted per vacuole. Na = not assessed. MEF = murine embryonic fibroblasts. BMDMs = Bone Marrow-Derived Macrophages. When not indicated, data from published works are from (7) and (115).

	Species	Phenotype *in vivo* (type *T. gondii*)	Cell system	Phenotype *in vitro* upon IFN-γ treatment (type *T. gondii*)		
				Host cell death [%]	*T. gondii* burden decrease [%]	*T. gondii* IC growth
Published work	*M. musculus* (inbred)	Resistance (II) Susceptible (I)	MEFs	~25 (II), 0 (I)	~ 50 (I), 90 (II)	na
			NIH/3T3 (111)	na	~80 (II)	na
			NIH/3T3 (182)	na	Decreased (I)	Unaffected (II)
	M. musculus castaneus	Resistance (I, II)	MEFs (CIM)	~ 25 (II and I)	~ 60 (I), 90 (II)	na
			CIM Δb2b1	na	~ 0 (I), na (II)	na
This study	*M. musculus*		Flp-In-3T3	~ 15 (I and II)	na	na
			Flp-BL6	~ 7 (I and II)	na	Decreased (II), Unaffected (I)
			Flp-CIM	~ 5 (I and II)	na	Decreased (II), Unaffected (I)

	Flp Δb2b1	~ 7 (I), 12 (II)	na	na
	Flp Δb2b1-BL6	~ 6 (I), 9 (II)	na	na
	Flp Δb2b1-CIM	~ 3 (I), 8 (II)	na	na
M. glareolus	BVK168	~20 (I), 2 (II)	na	Unaffected (I)
	BMDMs	~50 (I), 1 (II)	~40 (I, II)	Unaffected (I)
	Primary fibroblasts	~80 (I), 25 (II)	na	Unaffected (I)

Flp-In-3T3, and the derived Flp-CIM and Flp-BL6, do not mirror the phenotype displayed by murine fibroblast cultures in literature. The parental Flp-In-3T3 cells display an IFN-γ-mediated increase of ~15 % in necrotic cells compared to untreated controls during both type I and II *T. gondii* infection. Results on Flp-In-3T3 cells from Propidium Iodide (PI) stainings and from a preliminary cytotoxicity assay are in agreement (Fig. 16, Appendix Fig. 39). The necrotic death phenotype for type II infection is not to the extent of published data. First results obtained with the cytotoxicity assay, which uses the release of lactate dehydrogenase (LDH) from dying cells as proxy for cell death, made us questioning the validity of the assay and was not performed further. However, the PI-assay confirmed this phenotype. Surprisingly, the same proportion of dying cells was observed following type I infection, indicating that cells are not completely susceptible to the parasite (Fig. 16). The high concentration of mouse IFN-γ used (200 U/ml), chosen accordingly to previous studies (7), could account for this modest resistant phenotype during virulent infection. Indeed, already half of the IFN-γ concentration was shown to partially limit virulent parasite proliferation in murine inbred cells (7, 182). In our experiments IFN-γ was the only inducer of host immune response, since the main aim was the expression of *Irg* genes. However, during infection cells receive more stimuli and studies showed the importance of the TNF-α pathways' activation in parasite control, both in hematopoietic and not hematopoietic cells of mouse and human origin (74, 76, 200). The IFN-γ/TNF-α axis is not dispensable in parasite control (74), even though NIH/3T3 cells' control of virulent parasite does not significantly increase when stimulated with both cytokines (182).

As expected, since already the Flp-In-3T3 wt phenotype did not reproduce published results, Flp-BL6 and Flp-CIM did not either (Fig. 16). A lower percentage of positive control IFN-γ-treated Flp-CIM cells underwent cell death compared to the parental strain during parasite infection. Both cell lines did not display visible differences in parasite growth and preliminary counts of type I parasite number per vacuole confirmed no differences between Flp-BL6 and Flp-CIM cells (Appendix Fig. 38). Control of type II parasite intracellular growth was to the same extent in both cell lines (Appendix Fig. 38).

Flp-In-3T3 cells express an unexpectedly high amount of endogenous IRGb2-b1 (Fig. 17c), similarly to the parental strain NIH/3T3 (not shown) but much higher to what previously published on BL6 MEFs

(163). Establishment of a primary murine fibroblast culture confirmed the lower amount of IRGb2-b1 in primary cells compared to immortalized cell lines available to us (Fig. 17c). Since the amount of endogenous protein greatly exceeded the transfected one (Fig. 17a), I speculated that the two might interfere and directly cause the not reproducibility of the *T. gondii* infection phenotype in Flp-In-3T3 transfected cells. However, via creation of the knock-out cell line, Flp Δb2-b1, I proved that the endogenous protein is not influencing for the phenotype. Established Flp Δb2-b1-CIM and Flp Δb2-b1-BL6 cell lines displayed the same phenotype to *T. gondii* infection in a PI-assay as the cell lines with the endogenous *Irgb2-b1* (Fig. 18b). I concluded that this specific cell culture-based system cannot be used to study *Irg* genes since it does not reproduce the resistance phenotype for still unknown reasons. Unfortunately, Flp-In-3T3 cells were the only available murine cell type with the FRT cloning-based system. To still benefit of the produced plasmids and of the cloning strategy, production of different mouse cell systems with introduced FRT sequence is possible. To investigate bank vole IRGb2-b1-like role in resistance to *T. gondii*, we cloned *Irgb2-b1*$_{BVK}$ in CIM Δb2b1 via an alternative lentiviral system since both this cell line and protocol were established (115). Characterization of the *T. gondii* infection phenotype in this cell line is currently ongoing.

Because of the use of degenerated primers, the *Irgb2-b1* sequences we cloned in pES51-bl were all characterized by the presence of a myristoylation MGXXS sequence at the N-terminal (Fig. 7 and 9), which is signature of most murine effectors and decoy *Irg* genes (91). However, the original *Irgb-b1*$_{CIM}$ sequence has instead a MDXXS sequence that, because of our approach, was mutated into MGXXS, turning the protein into a putative target of myristoylation. The latter is a post-translational modification that facilitates membrane binding (83). Whether IRGs are target of myristoylation and the role of the modification on the protein function were never assessed. The mutated sequence was cloned in the Flp-CIM cell line first and in the Flp Δb2b1-CIM cell line after. We cannot exclude that this mutation was the direct cause of the not reproducibility of the resistance phenotype in created cell lines. However, *Mus musculus Irgb2-b1*$_{PWK/Ph}$ allele is also associated with resistance to virulent *T. gondii in vivo* and *in vitro* and has the myristoylation sequence in common with the susceptible *Irgb2-b1*$_{BL6}$ ((62), Catalina Alvarez personal communication). Of note if the presence of cysteines, which are target of palmitoylation, all throughout the sequence including the C-terminal which is a putative target site for this modification. Palmitoylation, similarly to myristoylation, facilitates protein membrane binding, as well as farnesylation which is a common modification of other small GTPases as Ras proteins (201). Post-translational modifications of IRG proteins in general, and of IRGb2-b1 in particular, warrant investigation and might shed light on their mechanism of actions which are still debated.

7.1.3 Expression levels of *Irg* genes in Flp-In-3T3 cells

Irgb2-b1 is highly expressed in resistant murine cell lines, i.e. *M. musculus castaneus* CIM and *M. musculus musculus* PWK/Ph (7), whereas specific residues associated with resistance are not clearly recognizable (Fig. 9). Thus, we can speculate that the expression level of resistant alleles might be another crucial factor in *Irg*-mediated resistance. *In vitro* systems where the expression of these genes can be easily controlled should be developed to define the importance of protein abundance over gene sequence. Promoters with different strength in gene expression can be assembled via Golden Gate in plasmids cloned with known resistant and susceptible *Irgb2-b1* genes and transfected in Flp-based systems. Studies on a natural population of voles already linked expression levels of different immune and not immune genes with susceptibility to different pathogens (202).

Excessive amounts of alleles have also been observed to cause the not reproducibility of resistance phenotype in expression cell systems. For example, overexpression of resistance-mediating *Irga6* unexpectedly led to an increased susceptibility *to C. trachomatis* in mouse cells (123). The authors speculated that the protein excess might interfere with other players in the host immune response and eventually reverse the phenotype. Similarly, the EF-1α promoter of choice to induce expression of introduced *Irg* sequences in Flp-In-3T3 cells is a strong promoter. We cannot exclude that non-physiological amounts of xenogenous resistant IRGb2-b1$_{CIM}$ hamper, instead of mediating, the host immune response. Low expression or polymorphisms in effectors *Irg* genes or other important mediators, like *Irga6* or *GBP2* necessary for its loading on the PVM (203), could also account for the lack of reproducibility of the infection phenotype in Flp-In-3T3 cells. *M. musculus castaneus* CAST/Ei cells express high levels of a resistance-associated *Irgb2-b1* allele but not of effector *Irg* genes, like *Irga6* and *Irgb6* (163). Nevertheless, CAST/Ei cells display the resistance phenotype to type I infection. Since host resistance is a result of all these immune players, having a complete picture of Flp-In-3T3 cell-autonomous mediators would help to interprete the infection outcome.

7.1.4 Genetic diversity of both laboratory host cells and parasites strains

In this study we address only the host genetic variability, keeping as constant the parasite background by using laboratory strains. However, it is well known that due to continue passaging, especially of the most commonly used RH strains, several mutations accumulated in the parasite genome resulting in strains highly different from early isolates (204). Laboratory strains adapted to *in vitro* cultures and are characterized by a higher extracellular survival, faster growth, formation of bigger plaques and inability to form orally infectious cysts. Additionally, they recruit less IRGa6 on the PVM and they are more resilient to host-mediated killing compared to fresh isolates (205). Thus, the use of laboratory-adapted virulent strains might contribute to the lack of reproducibility in our results. To properly address the hypothesis that wild rodents are resistant to virulent *T. gondii* strains *in vivo* and *in vitro*, fresh isolates should be used, which unfortunately are not easily accessible.

At the same time, a recent whole genome sequencing of 14 different stocks of one of the most diffused laboratory cell lines, the cervical cancer HeLa cells, revealed an enormous genetic diversity which contributes for sure to the current reproducibility crisis in the scientific community (206). These genetic differences were associated with different phenotype during infection with *Salmonella* (206). We cannot exclude the same happening for another largely diffused cell line, as the NIH/3T3 cells used in this study, during *T. gondii* infection. Furthermore, Flp-In-3T3 cell line could behave differently compared to parental NIH/3T3 cells, as already documented in a study where loss of multipotency was observed (207).

7.2 Role of non-murine wild rodents as reservoir for virulent *T. gondii*

7.2.1 Detection of *T. gondii* infection in wild rodents

Data collected in chapter 3.2.2 of the introduction indicate that non-murine species as *Microtus* spp., *M. glareolus* and *Apodemus* spp., have a higher *T. gondii* prevalence and are less susceptible to virulent parasite infection. Some considerations have to be added in this regard. There is currently no gold standard for assessing anti-*T. gondii* antibodies prevalence and chronic infection, and a systematic comparison of different diagnostic methods in terms of sensitivity and specificity has been performed only in few isolated cases (192, 208). This makes interpretation of results between different studies using different detection methods hazardous. The most used techniques include the Enzyme-Linked Immunosorbent Assay (ELISA) and the Modified Agglutination Test (MAT), the latter not relying on cross-reactivity of antibodies therefore of broader use. PCR amplification of specific parasite markers, even though necessary to assess the genotype, is currently less in use as diagnostic tool since it requires a DNA extraction step from bradyzoites. Differences in prevalence within the same rodent species could also be due to technical issues related to the test in use, e.g. not cross-reactivity of an antibody or less sensitivity of the technique. Finally, rats could be serologically negative even when they harbour *T. gondii* cysts (209) via still unclear mechanisms. This leads to underestimation of the prevalence rates and might happen for other rodent species as well.

Another factor influencing *T. gondii* prevalence data is the sampling. There is a positive correlation between rodent seroprevalence to *T. gondii* and proximity to human populated areas (210) where the probability of getting infected via cat feces is higher (211), as shown by studies in south France. Information regarding oocysts density, which might explain geographical seroprevalence heterogeneity, are scarce in Europe (212). Studies conducted in urban areas in UK and Senegal reported higher prevalences data than in rural areas (59, 192). Sampling might explain why *T. gondii* rodent positive samples were not identified in Germany in one study (18), whereas a more recent work in Berlin found a high percentage of infected rodents (49). In the latter all rodents trapped in woods where not infected with *T. gondii*, whereas prevalence was higher in the urban environment.

However, studies using different methods come to the same conclusion confirming non-murine spp. having higher *T. gondii* prevalence than *Mus* spp. in Europe. All mentioned variables bring even higher confidence to this assertion, which is further reinforced by the mentioned *in vivo* studies.

Concerning the present genotypes, most of the studies in literature genotype *T. gondii* on the basis of few, sometimes a single, genetic markers. The importance of an increased number of genetic markers is highlighted by the work from Schares et al. who re-classified German isolates as atypical instead of classic type II strains when using nine markers instead of the previously used four (183, 213). This result brings evidence to consider more reliable studies with a higher genetic resolution, even though less common. Studies in Europe describing virulent alleles in animal and human isolates on the basis of a single marker, mostly SAG2, should be expanded to investigate other markers (214-216). It has not been described so far whether certain within the 11 markers are more representative of genotype virulence than others, precluding the possibility of using a subset of them. The only molecular characterization with all the 11 markers in living voles – the Asiatic *Microtus fortis* – confirmed the high prevalence of *T. gondii* infection (53.8 %) and chronic infection with virulent genotypes (66, 67). This study supports the hypothesis that voles can be reservoir of virulent strains and European voles should be investigated further.

7.2.2 *T. gondii* infection of *M. glareolus* cells

7.2.2.1 *T. gondii* growth in *M. glareolus* cells

As reported in Tab. 20 and highlighted in pink, *M. glareolus* cells display a resistance phenotype to virulent parasite infection and decreased parasite burden following IFN-γ treatment (Fig. 32 and 34). This phenotype recalls *M. musculus castaneus* CIM cells during infection with both type I and II *T. gondii*. Similarly, I observe a drastic decrease in the population of living infected cells, which will further support dissemination. Despite a decrease in parasite burden, *T. gondii* intracellular growth in different *M. glareolus* cell types did not change following IFN-γ treatment (Fig. 31). A decrease in overall number of infected cells without affecting intracellular parasite growth was already reported in other studies (203). However, this phenotype is in contrast with results from the flow cytometry-based assay. In the latter the MFI was measured on the population of living infected cells and would imply an increase in vacuoles with only one or two parasites following IFN-γ treatment. Possible explanations are a) the higher number of cells analyzed per condition in the flow cytometry assay compared to the parasite counts (20,000 vs 100) which provides higher confidence in the results; b) an effect on the number of vacuoles per cell rather than number of parasites per vacuole.

Of note is that, despite use of the same parasite strain and amount, BVK168 cells support a higher virulent parasite growth compared to primary vole cells and murine cells (Fig. 31). The phenotype could be either cell type-specific or due to changes during the spontaneous immortalization (125). A difference between immortalized and primary kidney African green monkey cell cultures has been observed, but contrary to our results, primary monkey-derived cultures sustain higher *T. gondii* growth (174). A comparison with primary bank vole cells should be performed to allow interpretation of the phenotype.

Surprisingly, BVK168 cells infected with the virulent strain show an equal number of plaques following IFN-γ treatment, but of bigger size (Fig. 28b). This puzzling result made me consider different possible explanations. First, I observed that *T. gondii* blocks the STAT1-mediated pathway in vole cells when infection preceds the IFN-γ treatment, as demonstrated with the established reporter cell line (Fig. 29). It should be assessed whether the parasite is also able to block the pathway of IFN-γ stimulated cells. This blocking of the host immune response would explain the invariate number of plaques in the assay. The bigger plaque size could be explained by IFN-γ-induced premature egress of parasites from dying cells and infection of neighboring cells. The heavy infection of not necrotic cells in BVK168 cells and the decrease in live uninfected BMDMs compared to untreated control cells support this hypothesis (Fig. 32b and 34a). Induced egress of parasites is a conserved mechanism in human (150, 217) and mouse cells (105, 218), in the latter proved to happen *in vivo* via adoptive transfer (218). This phenomenon is directly triggered by immune cells, mostly macrophages, in a Ca^{2+}-dependent fashion in murine models (218) and by nitric oxide (NO) in human cells (217). Whether in one study the prematurely egressed parasites were observed to lose the capacity to invade human fibroblasts (150), others showed unchanged virulence both *in vitro* and *in vivo* (150, 217, 218). According to the model suggested by Tomita et al., premature egress is also a form of host resistance since it does not support parasite growth and increases the chance for IFN-γ-primed immune cells to mediate parasite killing and clear infection (218). It is easy to imagine that different cell types are present at the infection site, and freshly egressed parasites from kidney cells or fibroblasts can be phagocytized and killed by neighboring macrophages.

7.2.2.2 IFN-γ-dependant *M. glareolus* cell death following virulent *T. gondii* infection

M. glareolus cells undergo IFN-γ-mediated cell death when infected with type I but not type II strains, regardless of the cell type – i.e. kidney cell line, primary fibroblasts and BMDMs – as measured by the increase in Propidium Iodide stained nuclei (Fig. 32a). Phenotype in BMDMs was confirmed with a flow cytometry-based assay by using a fixable dye specific for dead cells (Fig. 34). A preliminary cytotoxicity assay performed on BVK168 cells confirmed the IFN-γ-dependent resistance phenotype (Appendix Fig. 39). Taken together, all results confirm that IFN-γ-treated *M. glareolus* cells die when infected with virulent *T. gondii*. Results from literature observed the infecting parasites to die within the dying cells (109). Therefore, host-killing was interpreted as defense mechanism.

Activation of the programmed cell death named pyroptosis has been documented in murine macrophages (109). However, a different cell death mechanism has been observed during type III infection (219). The hypothesis that a combination of different parasite strains and host cell types and species triggers different cell fate is a likely scenario. Type II *T. gondii* infection in *M. glareolus* BMDMs do not induce an increase in the amount of necrotic cells (Fig. 34). However, IFN-γ-treatment halves the amout of infected BMDMs and type II parasite burden (Fig. 34). The phenotype in vole BMDMs does not mirror what happens in *M. musculus* infection with medium virulent strains and might represent a novel mechanism of parasite control (109). These data do not exclude as well the possibility that *M. glareolus* is susceptible to type II T. gondii genotypes, similarly to other European mammals (220).

The use of rec*Tg*LEA protein as control proved that STAT1 signaling induction and subsequent expression of *Irg*-like genes are specifically induced by rec*Mg*IFN-γ (Fig. 24 and 27), and not by contaminants in the preparation. The displayed resistance phenotype during *T. gondii* infections on vole cells is IFN-γ-dependent, therefore not caused by possible contaminants. However, the latter could influence parasite replication and fitness and the experiments included only a control with untreated cells. Despite antiviral potency of rec*Mg*IFN-γ was shown to be strictly associated with the cytokine compound (Fig. 25), future infection experiments with *T. gondii* should include rec*Tg*LEA as control.

7.2.2.3 Expression of *Irg*-like genes in *M. glareolus* cells

M. glareolus parasite control during infection with both strains is dependant on type II cytokine stimulation. Despite a pool of IFN-γ-induced genes is expressed even in absence of the STAT1 transcriptional factor, the IRG family of protein in not within this class (171). Transcriptomic analysis in different inbred mouse cell types reports that *Irgb2-b1* is not highly expressed (Gene ID 620913) compared for example to another *Irg* gene like *Irga6* ((182), Gene ID 60440). Lilue et al. further confirmed this low *Irgb2-b1* expression in murine fibroblasts of susceptible mice (7). On the contrary, *Irgb2-b1* is highly expressed in fibroblast cells of resistant mouse strains, i.e. *M. musculus castaneus* CIM and *M. musculus musculus* PWK/Ph (7, 62). Preliminary data suggest that *Irgb2-b1*-like genes are not significantly induced following IFN-γ treatment in *M. glareolus* BMDMs and primary fibroblasts compared to untreated controls (not shown), whereas kidney cells show a 8-fold increase (Fig. 24). However, all cell types display a resistance phenotype to virulent parasite infection in an IFN-γ-dependant fashion. Surely *Irgb2-b1*-like mRNA abundance should be further assessed in these cell types in the future and the *Irgb2-b1*-like genes from primary cells sequenced. The RNAseq analysis currently ongoing will shed lights on the complete structure of the *Irg* family in these non-model organisms and serve as pioneering work for future sequence analysis.

Unfortunately, antibodies developed against murine IRG proteins do not cross-react with voles, likely due to differences in the recognized peptide sequences (Tab. 19). Therefore, a direct comparison between IRGb2-b1 protein in murine and vole cells via anti-IRGb2-b1 antibody is not possible (Fig. 35a). This lack of cross-reactivity precludes us to assess IRG protein loading directly in the wild rodents-derived cell lines. However, studies report contradictory results about correlations between PVM IRGs coating and parasite killing. Indeed, whereas resistant CIM-derived cells load IRG on almost all PVM compared to susceptible mice cells (7), parasites with coated vacuoles have been observed escaping the host cell (62, 221). Thus IRGs loading, even though providing information regarding host immune kinetic, is still a debated proxy for parasite killing.

7.2.2.4 Other resistance mechanisms to *T. gondii* infection in rodents

I do not exclude that IFN-γ-related mechanisms other that IRGs mediate *M. glareolus* resistance to parasite infection. Reactive oxygen species (ROS) and nitric oxide (NO) have been described to limit *T. gondii* growth in different species and cell types (77). Therefore, I performed a Griess assay to measure production of nitrite/nitrate (NO_2^-/NO_3^-), which are the final oxydative product of nitric oxide (NO), to assess the role of this mechanism in host resistance. I used the supernatant from *M. glareolus* BMDMs during the PI-assay in Fig. 32, where a resistant phenotype towards virulent parasites was observed. However, no detectable increase in the nitrite/nitrate ratio in vole BMDM was observed under any conditions, contrary to *Mus musculus* BMBDs treated with LPS used as positive control (Appendix Fig. 40). These results suggest that NO does not play a role in vole resistance to *T. gondii*, similarly to what observed in other studies on mice (74). However, the lack of phenotype could also be explained by a natural lower nitrite/nitrate ratio which reduces the possibility of NO_2^- detection, similarly to human cells.

Another recently identified family of IFN-γ-induced small GTPases, named GTPase IMmunity Associated Proteins (GIMAP), was associated with Lewis (LEW) rat resistance to virulent parasite infection compared to susceptible Brown Norway (BN) rats (222). Rats always constituted a classic animal model to study *T. gondii* (209) and are particularly suited to study susceptibility to infection since the mentioned common laboratory strains display opposite outcomes (223). GIMAPs localize at the PVM and restrict parasite growth via lysosomal fusion (222). However, the mechanism is cell-specific and takes place only in hematopoietic cells and not in intestinal epithelial cells, which highlights the importance of the cell types used in experiments. The role of IRGb2-b1-like proteins in LEW rat resistance to *T. gondii* is currently being investigated (Jeroen Saeij, personal communication). Until now, the major recognized mediator of resistance in LEW rats is the inflammasome sensor Nlrp1. Specific polymorphisms in the gene are conserved in all *T. gondii* refractory rat strains (224-226). Inflammasome activation eventually leads to host programmed cell death via pyroptosis. Similarly to rats, allelic variation of *Nlrp* orthologous loci accounts for species-specific inflammasome induction during *T. gondii* infection – and thus outcome – in laboratory mouse strains (227, 228) and human cells (229, 230). The other major family of GTPases involved in host defense to *T. gondii*, GBPs, regulates activation of the inflammasome (231). A regulation by IRG proteins deserves further investigation.

Finally, apart from the well-studied role of type II interferon, other IFN-γ-independent mechanisms appeared to play a critical role in *T. gondii* infection. For example IFN-ß response is activated in murine macrophages during infection with virulent atypical strains from South America and is associated with parasite killing independently of IFN-γ pathway activation (200). The importance of type I interferon pathway is also evident from the conserved parasite mechanisms directly evolved against it (90). The role of IFN-ß in different host species and cell types has not been addressed yet.

GIMAPs, inflammasome and IFN-ß pathways activation are just example of other defense mechanisms important in other *T. gondii* intermediate hosts and which impact during infection needs to be explored in voles.

7.3 New tools for research on non-model organisms

7.3.1 Production of a recombinant *M. glareolus* IFN-γ

The field of eco-immunology would greatly benefit from availability of still lacking immunological resources, such as cytokines, as already recognized by Zimmerman et al. (232). Here we provide the key recombinant *M. glareolus* IFN-γ cytokine, for which I demonstrated its activity not only on the same species, but also on a closely related vole species as *M. arvalis*. Availability of this cytokine allows addressing immunological responses of wild rodent cell lines *in vitro* during infection with pathogens that activate the type II interferon response. These include a multitude of bacteria, viruses and, as demonstrated here, intracellular parasites such as *T. gondii*.

RecMgIFN-γ was produced in high yield in *E. coli* and mostly in its active dimeric form of ca. 36 kDa. Detected proteins of different molecular weight were interpreted as monomeric, trimeric and higher order aggregates of the protein (Fig. 20). Such aggregates are known to occur with recIFN-γ under non-native conditions (233-236), as is e.g. the case during SDS-PAGE. The small 15 kDa protein not reactive with an anti-6His-tag antibody (Fig. 20a) was inconsistently observed in different preparations. A possible explanation is the bacterial strain of choice, OmniMax 2T1R, which provided better expression results compared to other strains, but which expresses the outer membrane protease OmpT (Steffen Zander, personal communication). This protease is known to cut within the C-terminal stretch of basic amino acids of *H. sapiens* IFN-γ (237, 238), resulting in the frequently observed truncated, but otherwise stable ca. 15-16 kDa IFN-γ (237, 239). We therefore assume that this protein is a C-terminal degradation product and is co-purified by dimer formation with a 6His-tagged monomer. Given the lack of availability of anti-vole IFN-γ antibodies which directly target the C-terminal stretch, only a mass spectrometry analysis of the protein suspension would validate this current hypothesis and might be performed in future studies.

Of note is the extended conserved C-terminal stretch in voles and human IFN-γ sequences, which is not present in murine species (Fig. 19b). Interestingly, C-terminal deletion mutants of recombinant human IFN-γ up to the basic stretch showed higher antiviral activity than the corresponding wild-type cytokine (239-242). This observation was attributed to a higher stability of the truncated protein (239). Another possible explanation is related to the recent work from Dufour et al. (243) who found an association between truncation in the C-terminal of human and murine IFN-γ and an anti-inflammatory mechanism. The cleavage happens in two sequential steps, the first targeting exactly the extended C-terminal which is shared between voles and human proteins, and the second upstream of the basic stretch. This finding indicates that this cleavage might take place in vole species as well, to activate specific immune pathways. However, a molecular mechanism, identification of the target of the truncated domain and information on whether differently conserved amino acids between species activate different pathways, are still missing. It is tempting to speculate that the extension beyond the basic stretch has evolved differently in different species to allow fine-tuning of the interaction between IFN-γ and its specific receptor molecules and thus cellular activation.

We show that recMgIFN-γ is active on other vole species than *M. glareolus*, like *M. arvalis*, likely due to sequence similarity. This cross-reactivity increases the applicability of this cytokine, which can be used to study the immunological response to pathogens in other rodents. For example, the zoonotic parasite *Babesia microti* is highly prevalent (up to 45 %) in European populations of *M. arvalis* (244) and causes basesiosis in humans with malaria-like symptoms (245). The genetic background of inbred mice has been shown to influence the phenotype to infection (246) and could be the reason behind contradictory results on the dispensability of IFN-γ during *B. microti* infection (247, 248). The provided recMgIFN-γ and a *M. arvalis*-derived cell line could shed light on the immune response to infection in the natural reservoir and provide a better background for epidemiological studies. Since *M. glareolus* shares more that 90 % of IFN-γ sequence homology with *M. agrestis* and *M. ochrogaster*, and 73.6 % with *Peromyscus maniculatus* (Fig. 19a), we hypothesize that rec*Mg*IFN-γ cross-reacts also with these other rodent species and its use in research can be extended even further.

I also observed that the commercial murine IFN-γ is active on *A. agrarius* cells (Fig. 21 and 23). An unusual dot-shaped nuclear signal of phospho-Ser727-STAT1 was observed in the *A. agrarius* AAL-R cell line compared to other vole and murine cells. The signal resembles the cytokine-induced paracrystalline forms of STAT3 observed by Droescher et al (249), which are more resilient to dephosphorylation and stay longer in an activated form. However, an association between this observation and the biological meaning was not further investigated. *Apodemus* spp. are more closely related to *Mus* spp. and are reservoirs of numerous pathogens (51). Many of the reagents already existing for the murine model can and should be validated for research on other *Muridae*. For example, preliminary results with an immunofluorescence assay applying anti-murine IRG antibodies showed a positive signal in *A. agrarius* cells (not shown), demonstrating the potential with that approach. However, the same assay did not return any reaction against *M. glareolus* (Tab. 20) and *M. arvalis* proteins (not shown).

Apart from type II interferon, we also report evidence of activity of the human hybrid type I interferon (IFN-αB/D) on bank vole cells (Fig. 25). Cross-activity of this cytokine was expected since type I interferon is less divergent than type II interferon and because activity of IFN-αB/D was already demonstrated in many and diverse mammalian species (144).

7.3.2 Establishment of *M. glareolus* in vitro systems

With the current work I established novel cell cultures of *M. glareolus*. In particular, I optimized protocols for differentiation of Bone Marrow-Derived Macrophages (BMDMs) and for the culturing of ear and tail-derived fibroblasts. Monocytes number increased significantly when a cocktail of both murine and human differentiating factors were used. This indicates that bank vole signalling pathways might share more identity with human than murine systems. This observation is also in line with other *M. glareolus*-derived cell culture-systems that were responsive to human factors (Estefania Delgado Betancourt, personal communication). The differentiated cells phenotypically resemble macrophages and display phagocytic capacity (Fig. 30a). However, the latter is not homogeneous in the culture which might indicate a not complete differentiation. Optimization of the differentiation protocol and further phenotypic characterization will be performed in the future. The observed polynucleated cells (Fig. 31d) can be residual megakaryocytes. This would explain the higher susceptibility to *T. gondii*. However, they appeared to increase in number following infection. Formation of multinucleated macrophages following *T. gondii* infection has been already observed in human macrophages (250). IFN-γ treatment is one of the main inducer of fusion, and the monocyte fusion capacity progressively decreases along with differentiation into macrophages (251). Formation of these giant cells has also been hypothesized to be an active defense process, with fresh monocytes fusing with infected macrophages to foster intracellular pathogen killing (251). Therefore, the big vacuoles present in multinucleated cells might contain parasites that display advantages and resist cellular killing.

The available BVK168 kidney cell line was already characterized and tested for susceptibility to different pathogens. To our knowledge we performed the first *in vitro* parasite infection in bank voles. BVK168 cells also proved to be easily transfectable with several transfection methods, which allowed me to establish the luciferase reporter cell line BVK-LucA. The most obvious use of BVK-LucA was to test rec*Mg*IFN-γ activity, as shown in Fig. 27. The non-linear dose-response with higher cytokine concentration (200 ng/ml) might be related to the recycling kinetics of the receptor subunit IFN-γR1, as reviewed before (79), or by IFN-γR1 expression inhibition via an autocrine-mediated loop following persistent activation as already observed for type I interferon (252). The observed maximal-fold induction of firefly luciferase in BVK-LucA cells is well in the range of values from other stable GAS-dependent luciferase-expressing cell lines reported in the literature (153, 252). The valuable role played by this cell line is not limited to test activity on IFN-γ. BVK-LucA cells can strengthen our knowledge around immune-modulation in vole cells, as we have shown by demonstrating *T. gondii* suppression of STAT1-mediated gene expression (Fig. 29). This suppression confirmed that the mechanism is not restricted to human and murine cells, but happens in *M. glareolus* cells as well. BVK-LucA cells can be used e.g. to test virus-specific defense mechanisms against host IFN-γ immune response. Variability in the antiviral assay with MHV68 (Fig. 25) and CPXV Brighton Red strain (not shown) might be due to evolution of specific virus mechanisms act at inhibiting this cytokine pathway, as already documented in these families of viruses (253, 254). Availability of the BVK-LucA cell line allows us to address this hypothesis. Cowpox and MHV68 viruses are considered highly species-specific, and different isolates result in opposite phenotypes in *in vivo* infection in voles (174, 177). This host-pathogen specificity can also account for variability in our *in vitro* viral experiments. Availability of an increasing number of wild rodents-derived cell lines and of established transfection protocols, allow us to establish more reporter cell lines to investigate cell type and species-specificity of pathogens. Gene-specific differences in sequence, length and spacing of the palindromic GAS sequences have been shown to contribute to its affinity for STAT1 (255). Thus, future analyses of vole genomes with regard to GAS elements of known, well-defined IFN-γ-regulated genes might lead to even more sensitive vole reporter cell lines.

7.3.3 Additional resources for research on *M. glareolus*

Apart from the provided different cell cultures and recombinant cytokine, with the current work I validated tools to address *in vitro* studies on bank voles. For example, I showed the usefulness of selected reagents developed for murine models, like antibodies specific for phosphorylated and not versions of STAT1 and for *β-actin*. The suitability of *Ywhaz* as housekeeping gene, which was published for *M. agrestis* (134), appeared solid for *M. glareolus* and *M. arvalis* as well (Fig. 24). Importantly, *β-Actin* was the least stable gene tested as housekeeping in *A. flavicollis* and hamsters (256-258), whereas is the most commonly used for *Mus musculus*. This highlights the importance of genomic references validation for each species, in order to avoid experimental artifacts, and is more and more frequently done in non-model organisms (57).

Another contribute to the field from our work is the RNAseq of BVK168 cells which is currently being analyzed and sums up to the other two bank vole transcriptomes available (see Tab. 21). Purpose for this RNAseq was to provide a complete map of expressed *Irg*-like genes in the three non-murine cell lines (in Tab. 16), which justifies the small set of samples. However, we do not exclude to increase in the future the number of samples for quantitative analysis if annotation results successful. Our RNAseq data include both IFN-γ-induced and not induced samples, which will provide for the first time the bank vole interferome.

The current work's impact on *M. glareoulus* research is obvious from Tab. 21, where the complete list of available reagents and references is reported.

Taken together, the tools provided with this project foster research on non-model animals as *M. glareolus* and *Microtus* spp.. Furthermore, preliminary results on voles' phenotype during *T. gondii* infection support their role as intermediate hosts for the parasite. This project paves the way to needed parasitological research in wildlife.

Tab. 21. Available resources for studies on *M. glareolus*.

	Description	**Source or reference**
Ear and tail primary fibroblasts		This work
BVK-LucA	Reporter cell line for IFN-γ activity	This work
BMDM	Bone Marrow Derived Macrophages	This work
rec*Mg*IFN-γ	Recombinant *M. glareolus* IFN-γ	This work
IFN-αB/D	Human hybrid type I interferon	(144), proved activity in this work.
Kidney transcriptome	RNAseq data of rec*Mg*IFN-γ-induced and not induced BVK168 cells	This work
Heart transcriptome		(259)
Liver transcriptome		(260)
Genome		GenBank 12837
BVK168 cell line	Kidney immortalized cell line	(125)
ES cells	Embryonic Stem cells	(261)
EF cells	Embryonic fibroblasts	(170)

8. Appendix

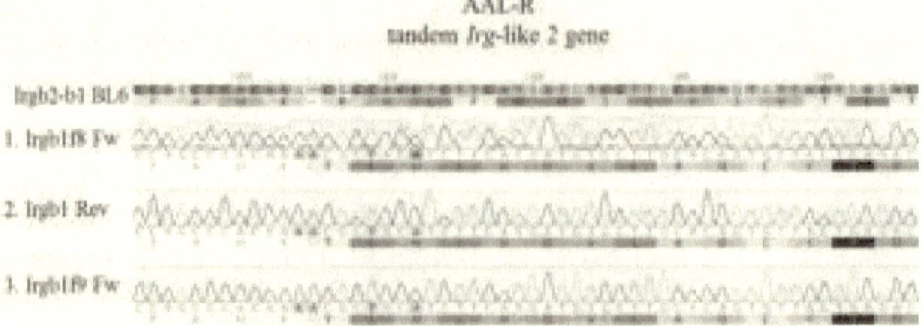

Appendix Fig. 37. Cloned AAL-R tandem 2 gene has stop codons in the *Irgb1*-like exon. Alignment of the cloned AAL-R tandem 2 *Irg*-like gene with *Irgb2-b1*$_{BL6}$. *Irgb2-b1*$_{BL6}$ was used as reference and nucleotide positions relative to the reference are indicated above. The cloned AAL-R tandem 2 *Irg*-like gene was sequenced with different primers (names reported on the left). Each sequence is reported with the nucleotide sequences and relative translation.

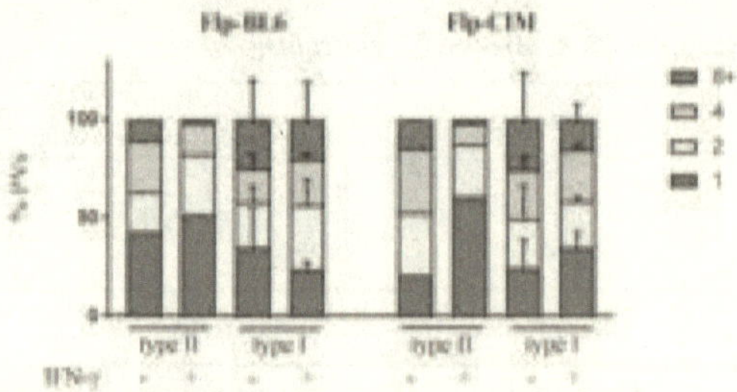

Appendix Fig. 38. Positive control Flp-CIM cell line does not display host resistance phenotype copared to negative control Flp-BL6. Negative control Flp-BL6 and positive control Flp-CIM cell lines were treated with 200 U/ml mouse IFN- γ or left untreated 24 h prior infection with avirulent (type II) and virulent (type I) *T. gondii*. 24 hpi cells were fixed and parasites per vacuole counted. Variance indicates that two independent experiments were performed.

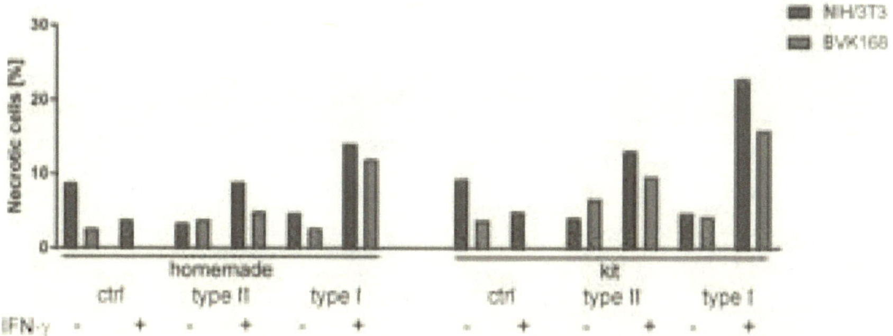

Appendix Fig. 39. Increase in necrotic cells following IFN-γ-treatment and virulent parasite infection in both in _M. glareolus_ and _M. musculus_ cells. Both _M. glareolus_ BVK168 cell line and murine NIH/3T3 cell line were treated with rec*Mg*IFN-γ (200 ng/ml) or mouse IFN-γ (200 U/ml) respectively, or left untreated as control 24 h prior infection with medium virulent (type II) and virulent (type I) _T. gondii_. 24 hpi the amount of extracellular LDH was measured at the Tecan reader as proxy for necrotic cell death. Absorbance values were normalized to the maximal LDH release of each cell line determined by full cell lysis. Both homemade reagents and a commercial kit were used. The experiment was performed once with 3 technical replicates.

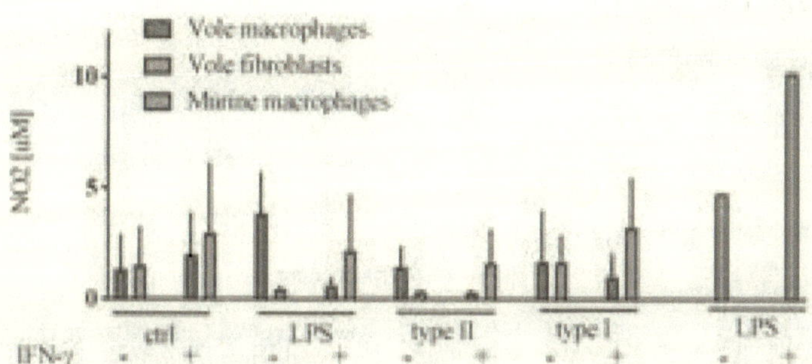

Appendix Fig. 40. _M. glareolus_ primary cells do not limit T. gondii proliferation via nitric oxyde. Griess assay to measure the amount of nitrite/nitrate (NO_2^-/NO_3^-) in solution, as indirect measure of nitric oxyde (NO) production. Vole cells (BMDMs and primary fibroblasts) were treated with rec*Mg*IFN-γ (200 ng/ml) and murine BMDMs with mouse IFN-γ (200 U/ml) or left untreated as control 24 h prior infection with medium virulent (type II) and virulent (type I) _T. gondii_. Treatment with LPS was used as positive control. Mean ± sd (n = 2 experiments, each with 2 replicates).

Tab. 21 Instrument list

Instrument	Company
2100 Bioanalyzer	Agilent Technologies Inc., CA, USA
ABI 7500 Real-Time PCR system	Applied Biosystem, Foster City, CA, USA
Accu-jet® pro pump	Brand GmbH, Wertheim, D
Äkta Purifier FPLC system	GE Healthcare, München, D
Agarose gel chambers *Mini-Sub® Cell GT System* and *Sub-Cell® GT System*	Bio-Rad Laboratories GmbH, München, D
Amaxa® Nucleofector® II Device	Lonza Cologne GmbH, Köln, D
Analytical balance A200S	Sartorius AG, Göttingen, D
Canon 450D	Canon Inc., Tokyo, Japan
Centrifuge Multifuge X1	Heraeus Holding GmbH, Hanau, D
Centrifuge Rotina 420R	Hettich LabTec, Tuttlingen, D
DNA-Workstation I	Kisker Biotech GmbH&Co. KG, Steinfurt, D
Electrophoretic gel chamber SDS Mini	Bio-rad Laboratories Inc., Hercules, CA, USA
Flow cytometer *CytoFLEX*	Beckman Coulter Inc., Brea, CA, USA
Gel documentation system	SERVA, Heidelberg, D
Gel documentation system Biometra TI-3	Biometra GmbH, Göttingen, D
Gel documentation system Universal Hood III	Bio-rad Laboratories Inc., Hercules, CA, USA
Heating block *Thermomixer compact*	Eppendorf AG, Hamburg, D
Hypoxia station Whitley H35	Meintrup DWS GmbH, Berlin, D
Incubator shaker *Innova®40*	New Brunswick Scientific, Edison, USA
Lightpad A930	Artograph Inc., Delano, MN, USA
Lumi-Imager	Peqlab Biotechnologie GmbH, Erlangen, D
Luminometer Tristar LB 941	Berthold Detection Systems GmbH, Pforzheim, D
Magnetic/Heating block *RCT basic IKAMAG®*	IKA Werke, Staufen, D
Microcentrifuge himac CT15RE	Hitachi Koki, Tokyo, Japan
Microcentrifuge Rotilabo®	Carl Roth GmbH & Co. KG, Karlsruhe, D

Instrument	Company
Microplate reader *Infinite® M200 PRO*	Tecan Group Ltd., Männedorf, Schweiz
Microscopes: AxioImager.Z1/ApoTome, AxioObserver.Z1 and confocal LSM780	Carl Zeiss GmbH, Jena, D
Microwave *Retro*	Melissa Classico, Skødstrup, D
Multichannel pipettes *Transferpette®-8/12*	Brand GmbH, Wertheim, D
pH Meter PB-11	Sartorius, Göttingen, D
Pipettes *Pipetman Classic™* 0.2-2 µL/ 1-10 µL/ 2-20 µL/ 50-200 µL/ 200-1,000 µL	Gilson Inc., Middleton, WI, USA
Pipette boy	Brand GmbH, Wertheim, D
Plate shaker	VWR International GmbH, Darmstadt, D
Power PAC 3000	Bio-Rad Laboratories GmbH, München, D
Precision balance TE1502S	Sartorius AG, Göttingen, D
Portable spectrophotometer *Ultrospec 10*	GE Healthcare, München, D
Safety Cabinet Series ASW-UP IV-1906	Bleymehl GmbH, Inden, D
Semi-dry membrane transfer system	Biometra GmbH, Göttingen, D
Spectrophotometer *NanoDrop® ND-1000*	Thermo Fisher Scientific Inc., Karlsruhe, D
Spectrophotometer *Quantus™ Fluorometer*	Promega GmbH, Madison, WI, USA
Sterilbank *Labgard Class II*	Integra Biosciences GmbH, Fernwald, D
Thermocycler *DNA Engine®*	Bio-Rad, München, D
Thermocycler *TPersonal*	Biometra GmbH, Göttingen, D
Transilluminator 470 nm	BioView Ltd., Billerica, USA
Ultrasonic bath Sonorex RK100H	BANDELIN electronic GmbH&Co.KG, Berlin, D
Vacuum pump *Mini-Vac power*	Peqlab Biotechnologie GmbH, Erlangen, D
Vortex-Genie® 2	Scientific Industries, New York, USA
Water bath GFL 1002	GFL mbH, Burgwedel, D

Tab. 22 Chemical list

Chemical	Company
Accutase Cell Detachment Solution	Capricorn Scientific GmbH, Ebsdorfergrund, D
Acetic acid 96 %	Merck KGaA, Darmstadt, D
Acrylamide 30 %	Sigma-Aldrich Chemie GmbH, Schnelldorf, D
Agarose	Biozym Scientific GmbH, Hessisch Oldendorf, D
Ammonium chloride	Sigma-Aldrich Chemie GmbH, Schnelldorf, D
Ammonium persulfate	Sigma-Aldrich Chemie GmbH, Schnelldorf, D
Amphotericin B	Capricorn Scientific GmbH, Ebsdorfergrund, D
Ampicillin	Carl Roth GmbH & Co. KG, Karlsruhe, D
Acetic acid 96 %	Merck KGaA, Darmstadt, D
ATP	Carl Roth GmbH & Co. KG, Karlsruhe, D
Bacto Tryptone	Carl Roth GmbH & Co. KG, Karlsruhe, D
Blasticidin	Invivo Gen, San Diego, CA, USA
β-mercaptoethanol	Carl Roth GmbH & Co. KG, Karlsruhe, D
Bromphenol blue	Merck KGaA, Darmstadt, D
BSA	Carl Roth GmbH & Co. KG, Karlsruhe, D
Calcium chloride	Carl Roth GmbH & Co. KG, Karlsruhe, D
CDTA	Sigma-Aldrich Chemie GmbH, Schnelldorf, D
Chloramphenicol	Sigma-Aldrich Chemie GmbH, Schnelldorf, D
Coenzyme A	Merck KGaA, Darmstadt, D
Collagenase type IV, CLS-4	Worthington Biochemical Corp., Lakewood, NJ, USA
Crystal violet	neoLab GmbH, Berlin, D
D(+)-Glucose	Sigma-Aldrich Chemie GmbH, Schnelldorf, D
DAPI	Sigma-Aldrich Chemie GmbH, Schnelldorf, D
Direct Blue (DB) 71	Sigma-Aldrich Chemie GmbH, Schnelldorf, D
D-Luciferin	Synchem UG&Co. KG Felsberg / Altenburg, D

Chemical	Company
DMEM high glucose (4.5 g/l) with sodium pyruvate and stable glutamine (GlutaMAX™)	ThermoFischer Scientific, Waltham, MA, USA
DMEM high glucose (4.5 g/l) without sodium pyruvate and phenol red, with stable L-glutamine	ThermoFischer Scientific, Waltham, MA, USA
DMEM high glucose (4.5g/l), with stable glutamine, with sodium pyruvate	Capricorn Scientific GmbH, Ebsdorfergrund, D
DMSO	Sigma-Aldrich Chemie GmbH, Schnelldorf, D
dNTPs	Carl Roth GmbH & Co. KG, Karlsruhe, D
Doxycycline hydrochloride	Fluka, Seelze, D
DTT	Carl Roth GmbH & Co. KG, Karlsruhe, D
EDTA	Carl Roth GmbH & Co. KG, Karlsruhe, D
Ethanol ≥ 99.5 %, pure or denatured with 1 % methyl ethyl ketone	Carl Roth GmbH & Co. KG, Karlsruhe, D
FCS	Sigma-Aldrich Chemie GmbH, Schnelldorf, D
Fluoromount™	Sigma-Aldrich Chemie GmbH, Schnelldorf, D
Formaldehyde	Carl Roth GmbH & Co. KG, Karlsruhe, D
GeneRuler™ 1 kb Plus DNA Ladder	Thermo Fisher Scientific Inc., Karlsruhe, D
Glycerol	Carl Roth GmbH & Co. KG, Karlsruhe, D
Glycine	Merck KGaA, Darmstadt, D
HEPES	Carl Roth GmbH & Co. KG, Karlsruhe, D
Hydrochloric acid	Carl Roth GmbH & Co. KG, Karlsruhe, D
Hygromycin B	Carl Roth GmbH & Co. KG, Karlsruhe, D
Hoechst 33342	Invitrogen™ Corporation, Carlsbad, CA, USA
human M-CSF	ImmunoTools GmbH, Friesoythe, D
Imidazole	Fluka, Seelze, D
Iodonitrotetrazolium chloride (INT)	Fluka, Seelze, D
IPTG	PEQLAB Biotechnologie GmbH, Erlangen, D

Chemical	Company
Isopropanol, pure	Carl Roth GmbH & Co. KG, Karlsruhe, D
Kanamycin	Carl Roth GmbH & Co. KG, Karlsruhe, D
Lactic acid	Sigma-Aldrich Chemie GmbH, Schnelldorf, D
Latex beads	Sigma-Aldrich Chemie GmbH, Schnelldorf, D
Lypopolysaccharide (LPS)	Sigma-Aldrich Chemie GmbH, Schnelldorf, D
Magnesium carbonate	Sigma-Aldrich Chemie GmbH, Schnelldorf, D
Magnesium chloride	Carl Roth GmbH & Co. KG, Karlsruhe, D
Magnesium sulfate	Merck KGaA, Darmstadt, D
Methanol, pure or *GC Ultra grade*	Carl Roth GmbH & Co. KG, Karlsruhe, D
MIDORI[Green] Direct nucleic acid stain	NIPPON Genetics Europe, Düren, D
Milk powder	Carl Roth GmbH & Co. KG, Karlsruhe, D
N-(1-Naphthyl)ethylenediamine	Sigma-Aldrich Chemie GmbH, Schnelldorf, D
NAD	SERVA Electrophoresis GmbH, Heidelberg, D
N-Methylphenazonium methyl sulfate	Fluka, Seelze, D
Sodium bicarbonate	Biochrom AG, Berlin, D
Sodium chloride	Carl Roth GmbH & Co. KG, Karlsruhe, D
Sodium citrate	Merck KGaA, Darmstadt, D
Sodium nitrate	Fluka, Seelze, D
Sulfanilamide	Sigma-Aldrich Chemie GmbH, Schnelldorf, D
Opti-MEM™ cell culture medium, Glutamax supplemented	ThermoFischer Scientific, Waltham, MA, USA
PageRuler Prestained Protein Ladder	ThermoFischer Scientific, Waltham, MA, USA
Paraformaldehyde	Carl Roth GmbH & Co. KG, Karlsruhe, D
Penicillin/Streptomycin (100 Units/100 µg pro mL; 100x)	Biochrom AG, Berlin, D
Phosphoric acid	Fluka, Seelze, D
PIPES	Carl Roth GmbH & Co. KG, Karlsruhe, D
Polyethylenimine (PEI) 25 KDa, linear	Polysciences Inc., Warrington, PA, USA

Chemical	Company
Potassium chloride	Carl Roth GmbH & Co. KG, Karlsruhe, D
Potassium phosphate dibasic	Merck KGaA, Darmstadt, D
Potassium phosphate monobasic	Merck KGaA, Darmstadt, D
Pronase E	Merck KGaA, Darmstadt, D
Propidium Iodide	Fluka, Seelze, D
Protease inhibitors: EDTA-free cOmplete™ Mini Protease Inhibitor Cocktail and PhosSTOP™	Sigma-Aldrich Chemie GmbH, Schnelldorf, D
Proteinase K	Carl Roth GmbH & Co. KG, Karlsruhe, D
Recombinant human M-CSF	ImmunoTools GmbH, Friesoythe, D
Recombinant mouse IFN-γ	Peprotech®, Rocky Hill, NJ, USA
RNaseZap™ RNase Decontamination Solution	ThermoFischer Scientific, Waltham, MA, USA
Sodium deoxycholate detergent	ThermoFischer Scientific, Waltham, MA, USA
SDS	Carl Roth GmbH & Co. KG, Karlsruhe, D
TEMED	Carl Roth GmbH & Co. KG, Karlsruhe, D
Timentin	Glaxo Smith Kline, London, UK
Tricine	Sigma-Aldrich Chemie GmbH, Schnelldorf, D
Tris	Merck KGaA, Darmstadt, D
Tris-Base	Carl Roth GmbH & Co. KG, Karlsruhe, D
Triton X-100	Fluka, Seelze, D
Trypsin/EDTA solution (10x)	Biochrom AG, Berlin, D
Tween-20	Merck KGaA, Darmstadt, D
X-Gal	Carl Roth GmbH & Co. KG, Karlsruhe, D
Yeast extract	Carl Roth GmbH & Co. KG, Karlsruhe, D

Consumables	Company
BRAND® 96-well deep well plates	Merck KGaA, Darmstadt, D
BRAND® mat cover for deep well plates	Merck KGaA, Darmstadt, D
C-Chip *Disposable Hemocytometer*	NanoEnTek Inc., Seoul, Korea
Cell culture flasks T25 / T75 / T150	TPP AG, Trasadingen, Schweiz
Cell scrapers	TPP AG, Trasadingen, Schweiz
Centrifuge tubes 15 und 50 ml	TPP AG, Trasadingen, Schweiz
Combitips	Eppendorf AG, Hamburg, D
Costar® low binding microcentrifuge tubes (0.65 and 1.7 ml)	Corning Inc., Corning, NY, USA
Coverslips (10 and 12 mm Ø)	VWR International GmbH, Darmstadt, D
Cuvettes Rotilabo®	Carl Roth GmbH & Co. KG, Karlsruhe, D
Inoculation loops	VWR International GmbH, Darmstadt, D
Microtiter plates 6/12/24/48/96-well	TPP AG, Trasadingen, CH
Microtiter µ-plate 96-well black	Ibidi GmbH, Planegg, D
Nitrocellulose membrane	GE Healthcare, München, D
Parafilm®	Pechiney Plastic Packaging, Chicago, IL, USA
Pasteur pipettes, 3 ml	VWR International GmbH, Darmstadt, D
Petri dishes 94x16 mm, steril	Carl Roth GmbH & Co. KG, Karlsruhe, D
Polycarbonate 3 µm filters	Whatman, Maidstone, UK
Serological pipettes	TPP AG, Trasadingen, CH
Slides 76x26 mm	Carl Roth GmbH & Co. KG, Karlsruhe, D
Syringes *Omnifix®* 5 / 10 / 20 ml	B. Braun Melsungen AG, Melsungen, D
Syringe filters *Minisart* 0.2 / 0.45 / 0.7 µm	Sartorius AG, Göttingen, D
Vacuum Midisart™ 2000 filters	Sartorius GmbH, Göttingen, D
Reaction tubes 0.5/1.5 ml	VWR International GmbH
Whatman paper	Carl Roth GmbH & Co. KG, Karlsruhe, D

9. References

1.   Nicolle C, Manceaux LH. On a leishman body infection (or related organisms) of the gondi. 1908. Int J Parasitol. 2009;39(8):863-4.
2.   Rougier S, Montoya JG, Peyron F. Lifelong Persistence of *Toxoplasma* Cysts: A Questionable Dogma? Trends Parasitol. 2017;33(2):93-101.
3.   Dubey JP. Toxoplasmosis of animals and humans: CRC press; 2016.
4.   Pappas G, Roussos N, Falagas ME. Toxoplasmosis snapshots: global status of *Toxoplasma gondii* seroprevalence and implications for pregnancy and congenital toxoplasmosis. Int J Parasitol. 2009;39(12):1385-94.
5.   Wilking H, Thamm M, Stark K, Aebischer T, Seeber F. Prevalence, incidence estimations, and risk factors of *Toxoplasma gondii* infection in Germany: a representative, cross-sectional, serological study. Sci Rep. 2016;6:22551.
6.   Clough B, Frickel EM. The *Toxoplasma* Parasitophorous Vacuole: An Evolving Host-Parasite Frontier. Trends Parasitol. 2017;33(6):473-88.
7.   Lilue J, Muller UB, Steinfeldt T, Howard JC. Reciprocal virulence and resistance polymorphism in the relationship between *Toxoplasma gondii* and the house mouse. Elife. 2013;2:e01298.
8.   English ED, Adomako-Ankomah Y, Boyle JP. Secreted effectors in *Toxoplasma gondii* and related species: determinants of host range and pathogenesis? Parasite Immunol. 2015;37(3):127-40.
9.   Howe DK, Sibley LD. Toxoplasma gondii comprises three clonal lineages: correlation of parasite genotype with human disease. J Infect Dis. 1995;172(6):1561-6.
10.   Dubey JP, Velmurugan GV, Rajendran C, Yabsley MJ, Thomas NJ, Beckmen KB, et al. Genetic characterisation of *Toxoplasma gondii* in wildlife from North America revealed widespread and high prevalence of the fourth clonal type. Int J Parasitol. 2011;41(11):1139-47.
11.   Khan A, Taylor S, Ajioka JW, Rosenthal BM, Sibley LD. Selection at a single locus leads to widespread expansion of *Toxoplasma gondii* lineages that are virulent in mice. PLoS Genet. 2009;5(3):e1000404.
12.   Shwab EK, Zhu XQ, Majumdar D, Pena HF, Gennari SM, Dubey JP, et al. Geographical patterns of *Toxoplasma gondii* genetic diversity revealed by multilocus PCR-RFLP genotyping. Parasitology. 2014;141(4):453-61.
13.   Chicaybam L, Sodre AL, Curzio BA, Bonamino MH. An efficient low cost method for gene transfer to T lymphocytes. PLoS One. 2013;8(3):e60298.
14.   Su C, Khan A, Zhou P, Majumdar D, Ajzenberg D, Darde ML, et al. Globally diverse *Toxoplasma gondii* isolates comprise six major clades originating from a small number of distinct ancestral lineages. Proc Natl Acad Sci U S A. 2012;109(15):5844-9.
15.   ToxoDB Toxoplama Genomics Resource.
16.   Ajzenberg D, Collinet F, Mercier A, Vignoles P, Darde ML. Genotyping of *Toxoplasma gondii* isolates with 15 microsatellite markers in a single multiplex PCR assay. J Clin Microbiol. 2010;48(12):4641-5.
17.   Su C, Shwab EK, Zhou P, Zhu XQ, Dubey JP. Moving towards an integrated approach to molecular detection and identification of *Toxoplasma gondii*. Parasitology. 2010;137(1):1-11.
18.   Herrmann DC, Maksimov P, Maksimov A, Sutor A, Schwarz S, Jaschke W, et al. *Toxoplasma gondii* in foxes and rodents from the German Federal States of Brandenburg and Saxony-Anhalt: seroprevalence and genotypes. Vet Parasitol. 2012;185(2-4):78-85.
19.   Verma SK, Ajzenberg D, Rivera-Sanchez A, Su C, Dubey JP. Genetic characterization of *Toxoplasma gondii* isolates from Portugal, Austria and Israel reveals higher genetic variability within the type II lineage. Parasitology. 2015;142(07):948-57.

20.   Jokelainen P, Murat JB, Nielsen HV. Direct genetic characterization of *Toxoplasma gondii* from clinical samples from Denmark: not only genotypes II and III. Eur J Clin Microbiol Infect Dis. 2018;37(3):579-86.

21.   Sroka J, Bilska-Zajac E, Wojcik-Fatla A, Zajac V, Dutkiewicz J, Karamon J, et al. Detection and molecular characteristics of *Toxoplasma gondii* DNA in retail raw meat products in Poland. Foodborne Pathog Dis. 2018.

22.   Boothroyd JC, Grigg ME. Population biology of *Toxoplasma gondii* and its relevance to human infection: do different strains cause different disease? Curr Opin Microbiol. 2002;5(4):438-42.

23.   Saraf P, Shwab EK, Dubey JP, Su C. On the determination of *Toxoplasma gondii* virulence in mice. Exp Parasitol. 2017;174:25-30.

24.   Su C, Howe DK, Dubey JP, Ajioka JW, Sibley LD. Identification of quantitative trait loci controlling acute virulence in *Toxoplasma gondii*. Proc Natl Acad Sci U S A. 2002;99(16):10753-8.

25.   Taylor S, Barragan A, Su C, Fux B, Fentress SJ, Tang K, et al. A secreted serine-threonine kinase determines virulence in the eukaryotic pathogen *Toxoplasma gondii*. Science. 2006;314(5806):1776-80.

26.   Saeij JP, Boyle JP, Coller S, Taylor S, Sibley LD, Brooke-Powell ET, et al. Polymorphic secreted kinases are key virulence factors in toxoplasmosis. Science. 2006;314(5806):1780-3.

27.   Reese ML, Zeiner GM, Saeij JP, Boothroyd JC, Boyle JP. Polymorphic family of injected pseudokinases is paramount in *Toxoplasma* virulence. Proc Natl Acad Sci U S A. 2011;108(23):9625-30.

28.   Behnke MS, Khan A, Wootton JC, Dubey JP, Tang K, Sibley LD. Virulence differences in *Toxoplasma* mediated by amplification of a family of polymorphic pseudokinases. Proc Natl Acad Sci U S A. 2011;108(23):9631-6.

29.   Shwab EK, Jiang T, Pena HF, Gennari SM, Dubey JP, Su C. The ROP18 and ROP5 gene allele types are highly predictive of virulence in mice across globally distributed strains of *Toxoplasma gondii*. Int J Parasitol. 2016;46(2):141-6.

30.   Etheridge RD, Alaganan A, Tang K, Lou HJ, Turk BE, Sibley LD. The *Toxoplasma* pseudokinase ROP5 forms complexes with ROP18 and ROP17 kinases that synergize to control acute virulence in mice. Cell Host Microbe. 2014;15(5):537-50.

31.   Lorenzi H, Khan A, Behnke MS, Namasivayam S, Swapna LS, Hadjithomas M, et al. Local admixture of amplified and diversified secreted pathogenesis determinants shapes mosaic Toxoplasma gondii genomes. Nat Commun. 2016;7:10147.

32.   Hakimi MA, Olias P, Sibley LD. *Toxoplasma* Effectors Targeting Host Signaling and Transcription. Clin Microbiol Rev. 2017;30(3):615-45.

33.   Yamamoto M, Ma JS, Mueller C, Kamiyama N, Saiga H, Kubo E, et al. ATF6beta is a host cellular target of the *Toxoplasma gondii* virulence factor ROP18. J Exp Med. 2011;208(7):1533-46.

34.   An R, Tang Y, Chen L, Cai H, Lai D-H, Liu K, et al. Encephalitis is mediated by ROP18 of *Toxoplasma gondii*, a severe pathogen in AIDS patients. Proc Natl Acad Sci U S A. 2018;115(23):E5344-E52.

35.   Powell CC, Lappin MR. Clinical ocular toxoplasmosis in neonatal kittens. Vet Ophthalmol. 2001;4(2):87-92.

36.   Dubey JP. Comparative infectivity of oocysts and bradyzoites of *Toxoplasma gondii* for intermediate (mice) and definitive (cats) hosts. Vet Parasitol. 2006;140(1-2):69-75.

37.   Zulpo DL, Sammi AS, Dos Santos JR, Sasse JP, Martins TA, Minutti AF, et al. *Toxoplasma gondii*: A study of oocyst re-shedding in domestic cats. Vet Parasitol. 2018;249:17-20.

38.   Turner DC, Bateson P, Bateson PPG. The Domestic Cat: The Biology of Its Behaviour: Cambridge University Press; 2000.
39.   Kitts-Morgan SE. Companion Animals Symposium: Sustainable Ecosystems: Domestic cats and their effect on wildlife populations. J Animal Sci. 2015;93(3):848-59.
40.   Széles GL, Purger JJ, Molnár T, Lanszki J. Comparative analysis of the diet of feral and house cats and wildcat in Europe. Mammal Research. 2017;63(1):43-53.
41.   Forin-Wiart MA, Poulle ML, Piry S, Cosson JF, Larose C, Galan M. Evaluating metabarcoding to analyse diet composition of species foraging in anthropogenic landscapes using Ion Torrent and Illumina sequencing. Sci Rep. 2018;8(1):17091.
42.   Biró Z, Lanszki J, Szemethy L, Heltai M, Randi E. Feeding habits of feral domestic cats (*Felis catus*), wild cats (*Felis silvestris*) and their hybrids: trophic niche overlap among cat groups in Hungary. J Zool. 2005;266(2):187-96.
43.   Germain E, Ruette S, Poulle M-L. Likeness between the food habits of European wildcats, domestic cats and their hybrids in France. Mamm Biol. 2009;74(5):412-7.
44.   Apostolico F, Vercillo F, La Porta G, Ragni B. Long-term changes in diet and trophic niche of the European wildcat (*Felis silvestris silvestris*) in Italy. Mammal Research. 2015;61(2):109-19.
45.   Sarmento P. Feeding ecology of the European wildcat *Felis silvestris* in Portugal. Acta Theriol. 1996;41(4):409-14.
46.   Woods MM, RA; Harris, S. Domestic Cat Predation on Wildlife. The Mammal Society; 2003.
47.   Tryjanowski P, Antczak M, Hromada M, Kuczynski L, Skoracki M. Winter feeding ecology of male and female European wildcats *Felis silvestris* in Slovakia. Eur J Wildl Res. 2002;48(1):49-54.
48.   IUCN red list of threatened species and the mammal society [Available from: https://www.iucn.org/iucn-red-list-threatened-species-test-single-page.]
49.   Krucken J, Blumke J, Maaz D, Demeler J, Ramunke S, Antolova D, et al. Small rodents as paratenic or intermediate hosts of carnivore parasites in Berlin, Germany. PLoS One. 2017;12(3):e0172829.
50.   Perec-Matysiak A, Bunkowska-Gawlik K, Zalesny G, Hildebrand J. Small rodents as reservoirs of *Cryptosporidium* spp. and *Giardia* spp. in south-western Poland. Ann Agric Environ Med. 2015;22(1):1-5.
51.   Schmidt S, Essbauer SS, Mayer-Scholl A, Poppert S, Schmidt-Chanasit J, Klempa B, et al. Multiple infections of rodents with zoonotic pathogens in Austria. Vector Borne Zoonotic Dis. 2014;14(7):467-75.
52.   Kilonzo C, Li X, Vivas EJ, Jay-Russell MT, Fernandez KL, Atwill ER. Fecal shedding of zoonotic food-borne pathogens by wild rodents in a major agricultural region of the central California coast. Appl Environ Microbiol. 2013;79(20):6337-44.
53.   Obiegala A, Woll D, Karnath C, Silaghi C, Schex S, Essbauer S, et al. Prevalence and genotype allocation of pathogenic *Leptospira* species in small mammals from various habitat types in Germany. PLoS Negl Trop Dis. 2016;10(3):e0004501.
54.   Yabsley MJ, Shock BC. Natural history of zoonotic *Babesia*: Role of wildlife reservoirs. Int J Parasitol Parasites Wildl. 2013;2:18-31.
55.   Tadin A, Tokarz R, Markotic A, Margaletic J, Turk N, Habus J, et al. Molecular survey of zoonotic agents in rodents and other small mammals in Croatia. Am J Trop Med Hyg. 2016;94(2):466-73.
56.   Ermonval M, Baychelier F, Tordo N. What Do We Know about How Hantaviruses Interact with Their Different Hosts? Viruses. 2016;8(8).
57.   Pedersen AB, Babayan SA. Wild immunology. Mol Ecol. 2011;20(5):872-80.

58.	Ehret T, Torelli F, Klotz C, Pedersen AB, Seeber F. Translational rodent models for research on parasitic protozoa-A review of confounders and possibilities. Front Cell Infect Microbiol. 2017;7:238.

59.	Murphy RG, Williams RH, Hughes JM, Hide G, Ford NJ, Oldbury DJ. The urban house mouse (*Mus domesticus*) as a reservoir of infection for the human parasite *Toxoplasma gondii*: an unrecognised public health issue? Int J Environ Heal R. 2008;18(3):177-85.

60.	Hide G, Morley EK, Hughes JM, Gerwash O, Elmahaishi MS, Elmahaishi KH, et al. Evidence for high levels of vertical transmission in *Toxoplasma gondii*. Parasitology. 2009;136(14):1877-85.

61.	Bajnok J, Boyce K, Rogan MT, Craig PS, Lun ZR, Hide G. Prevalence of *Toxoplasma gondii* in localized populations of *Apodemus sylvaticus* is linked to population genotype not to population location. Parasitology. 2015;142(5):680-90.

62.	Hassan MA, Olijnik AA, Frickel EM, Saeij JP. Clonal and atypical *Toxoplasma* strain differences in virulence vary with mouse sub-species. Int J Parasitol. 2018.

63.	Dymon M, Starzyk J, Slowakiewicz E, Pavlik B. Toxoplasmosis in small wild mammals occurring in southern Poland 1976.

64.	Starzyk J, Pawlik B, Dymon M. Investigations on the sensitivity of small wild mammals to the development of infection by *Toxoplasma gondii*. ACTA BIOL CRACOV. 1970;13.

65.	Fujii H, Kamiyama T, Hagiwara T. Species and strain differences in sensitivity to *Toxoplasma* infection among laboratory rodents. Jpn J Med Sci Biol. 1983;36:343-6.

66.	Zhang XX, Huang SY, Zhang YG, Zhang Y, Zhu XQ, Liu Q. First report of genotyping of *Toxoplasma gondii* in free-living *Microtus fortis* in northeastern China. J Parasitol. 2014;100(5):692-4.

67.	Zhang XX, Lou ZZ, Huang SY, Zhou DH, Jia WZ, Su C, et al. Genetic characterization of *Toxoplasma gondii* from Qinghai vole, Plateau pika and Tibetan ground-tit on the Qinghai-Tibet Plateau, China. Parasit Vectors. 2013;6:291.

68.	Hejlícek K, Literák I, Nezval J. Toxoplasmosis in wild mammals from the Czech Republic. Folia Zool. 1998;33(3):480-5.

69.	Doby JM, Demsmonts G, Beaucournu JC, Akinchina GT. Recherce immunologique systematique de la Toxoplasmose chez les petits mammiferes sauvages en France. Folia Parasitol. 1974;21:289-300.

70.	Meerburg BG, De Craeye S, Dierick K, Kijlstra A. *Neospora caninum* and *Toxoplasma gondii* in brain tissue of feral rodents and insectivores caught on farms in the Netherlands. Vet Parasitol. 2012;184(2-4):317-20.

71.	Jackson MH, Hutchison WM, Siim JC. Toxoplasmosis in a wild rodent population of central Scotland and a possible explanation of the mode of transmission. J Zool Lond. 1986;209(4):549-57.

72.	Delgado Betancourt E, Hamid B, Fabian BT, Klotz C, Hartmann S, Seeber F. From entry to early dissemination-*Toxoplasma gondii*'s initial encounter with its host. Front Cell Infect Microbiol. 2019;9:46.

73.	Scharton-Kersten TM, Wynn TA, Denkers EY, Bala S, Grunvald E, Hieny S, et al. In the absence of endogenous IFN- γ, mice develop unimpaired IL-12 responses to *Toxoplasma gondii* while failing to control acute infection. J Immunol. 1996;157(9):4045-54.

74.	Yap GS, Sher A. Effector cells of both nonhemopoietic and hemopoietic origin are required for interferon (IFN)-gamma- and tumor necrosis factor (TNF)-alpha-dependent host resistance to the intracellular pathogen, *Toxoplasma gondii*. J Exp Med. 1999;189(7):1083-92.

75.	Suzuki Y, Orellana MA, Schreiber RD, Remington JS. Interferon-gamma: the major mediator of resistance against *Toxoplasma gondii*. Science. 1988;240(4851):516-8.

76. Ceravolo IP, Chaves AC, Bonjardim CA, Sibley D, Romanha AJ, Gazzinelli RT. Replication of *Toxoplasma gondii*, but not *Trypanosoma cruzi*, is regulated in human fibroblasts activated with gamma interferon: requirement of a functional JAK/STAT pathway. IAI. 1999;67(5):2233-40.

77. Hunter CA, Sibley LD. Modulation of innate immunity by *Toxoplasma gondii* virulence effectors. Nat Rev Microbiol. 2012;10(11):766-78.

78. Safronova A, Araujo A, Camanzo ET, Moon TJ, Elliott MR, Beiting DP, et al. Alarmin S100A11 initiates a chemokine response to the human pathogen *Toxoplasma gondii*. Nat Immunol. 2019;20(1):64-72.

79. de Weerd NA, Nguyen T. The interferons and their receptors--distribution and regulation. Immunol Cell Biol. 2012;90(5):483-91.

80. Wen Z, Zhong Z, Darnell JE, Jr. Maximal activation of transcription by Stat1 and Stat3 requires both tyrosine and serine phosphorylation. Cell. 1995;82(2):241-50.

81. Hu X, Ivashkiv LB. Cross-regulation of signaling pathways by interferon-gamma: implications for immune responses and autoimmune diseases. Immunity. 2009;31(4):539-50.

82. Rusinova I, Forster S, Yu S, Kannan A, Masse M, Cumming H, et al. Interferome v2.0: an updated database of annotated interferon-regulated genes. Nucleic Acids Res. 2013;41(Database issue):D1040-6.

83. Boehm U, Guethlein L, Klamp T, Ozbek K, Schaub A, Futterer A, et al. Two families of GTPases dominate the complex cellular response to IFN-γ. J Immunol. 1998;161(12):6715-23.

84. MacMicking JD. Interferon-inducible effector mechanisms in cell-autonomous immunity. Nat Rev Immunol. 2012;12(5):367-82.

85. Kim BH, Shenoy AR, Kumar P, Bradfield CJ, MacMicking JD. IFN-inducible GTPases in host cell defense. Cell Host Microbe. 2012;12(4):432-44.

86. Rosowski EE, Saeij JP. *Toxoplasma gondii* clonal strains all inhibit STAT1 transcriptional activity but polymorphic effectors differentially modulate IFN-γ induced gene expression and STAT1 phosphorylation. PLoS One. 2012;7(12):e51448.

87. Gay G, Braun L, Brenier-Pinchart MP, Vollaire J, Josserand V, Bertini RL, et al. *Toxoplasma gondii* TgIST co-opts host chromatin repressors dampening STAT1-dependent gene regulation and IFN-γ-mediated host defenses. J Exp Med. 2016;213(9):1779-98.

88. Olias P, Etheridge RD, Zhang Y, Holtzman MJ, Sibley LD. *Toxoplasma* Effector Recruits the Mi-2/NuRD Complex to Repress STAT1 Transcription and Block IFN-γ-Dependent Gene Expression. Cell Host Microbe. 2016;20(1):72-82.

89. Nast R, Staab J, Meyer T, Luder CGK. *Toxoplasma gondii* stabilises tetrameric complexes of tyrosine-phosphorylated signal transducer and activator of transcription-1 and leads to its sustained and promiscuous DNA binding. Cell Microbiol. 2018;20(11):e12887.

90. Rosowski EE, Nguyen QP, Camejo A, Spooner E, Saeij JP. *Toxoplasma gondii* Inhibits gamma interferon (IFN-γ)- and IFN-β-induced host cell STAT1 transcriptional activity by increasing the association of STAT1 with DNA. IAI. 2014;82(2):706-19.

91. Bekpen C, Hunn JP, Rohde C, Parvanova I, Guethlein L, Dunn DM, et al. The interferon-inducible p47 (IRG) GTPases in vertebrates: loss of the cell autonomous resistance mechanism in the human lineage. Genome Biol. 2005;6(11):R92.

92. Muller UB, Howard JC. The impact of *Toxoplasma gondii* on the mammalian genome. Curr Opin Microbiol. 2016;32:19-25.

93. Coers J, Bernstein-Hanley I, Grotsky D, Parvanova I, Howard JC, Taylor GA, et al. *Chlamydia muridarum* evades growth restriction by the IFN-γ-Inducible Host Resistance Factor Irgb10. J Immunol. 2008;180(9):6237-45.

94.   Collazo CM, Yap GS, Sempowski GD, Lusby KC, Tessarollo L, Vande Woude GF, et al. Inactivation of LRG-47 and IRG-47 reveals a family of interferon gamma-inducible genes with essential, pathogen-specific roles in resistance to infection. J Exp Med. 2001;194(2):181-8.

95.   Henry SC, Daniell X, Indaram M, Whitesides JF, Sempowski GD, Howell D, et al. Impaired macrophage function underscores susceptibility to *Salmonella* in mice lacking Irgm1 (LRG-47). J Immunol. 2007;179(10):6963-72.

96.   Henry SC, Daniell XG, Burroughs AR, Indaram M, Howell DN, Coers J, et al. Balance of Irgm protein activities determines IFN-γ-induced host defense. J Leukoc Biol. 2009;85(5):877-85.

97.   Hunn JP, Feng CG, Sher A, Howard JC. The immunity-related GTPases in mammals: a fast-evolving cell-autonomous resistance system against intracellular pathogens. Mamm Genome. 2011;22(1-2):43-54.

98.   Ferreira-da-Silva Mda F, Springer-Frauenhoff HM, Bohne W, Howard JC. Identification of the microsporidian *Encephalitozoon cuniculi* as a new target of the IFN-γ-inducible IRG resistance system. PLoS Pathog. 2014;10(10):e1004449.

99.   MacMicking JD, Taylor GA, McKinney JD. Immune control of tuberculosis by IFN-γ-inducible LRG-47. Science. 2003;302(5645):654-9.

100.   Shi Y, Shen S, Hu S, Ding T, Hong X, Chen C, et al. Comparative study of two immunity-related GTPase genes in Chinese soft-shell turtle reveals their molecular characteristics and functional activity in immune defense. Dev Comp Immunol. 2018;81:63-73.

101.   Ghosh A, Uthaiah R, Howard J, Herrmann C, Wolf E. Crystal structure of IIGP1: a paradigm for interferon-inducible p47 resistance GTPases. Mol Cell. 2004;15(5):727-39.

102.   Mehto S, Jena KK, Nath P, Chauhan S, Kolapalli SP, Das SK, et al. The Crohn's disease risk factor IRGM limits NLRP3 inflammasome activation by impeding its assembly and by mediating its selective autophagy. Mol Cell. 2018.

103.   Maric-Biresev J, Hunn JP, Krut O, Helms JB, Martens S, Howard JC. Loss of the interferon-γ-inducible regulatory immunity-related GTPase (IRG), Irgm1, causes activation of effector IRG proteins on lysosomes, damaging lysosomal function and predicting the dramatic susceptibility of Irgm1-deficient mice to infection. BMC Biol. 2016;14:33.

104.   Taylor GA, Collazo CM, Yap GS, Nguyen K, Gregorio TA, Taylor LS, et al. Pathogen-specific loss of host resistance in mice lacking the IFN-γ-inducible gene IGTP. Proc Natl Acad Sci U S A. 2000;97(2):751-5.

105.   Melzer T, Duffy A, Weiss LM, Halonen SK. The gamma interferon (IFN-γ)-inducible GTP-binding protein IGTP is necessary for toxoplasma vacuolar disruption and induces parasite egression in IFN-γ-stimulated astrocytes. IAI. 2008;76(11):4883-94.

106.   Martens S, Sabel K, Lange R, Uthaiah R, Wolf E, Howard JC. Mechanisms regulating the positioning of mouse p47 resistance GTPases LRG-47 and IIGP1 on cellular membranes: retargeting to plasma membrane induced by phagocytosis. J Immunol. 2004;173(4):2594-606.

107.   Papic N, Hunn JP, Pawlowski N, Zerrahn J, Howard JC. Inactive and active states of the interferon-inducible resistance GTPase, Irga6, in vivo. J Biol Chem. 2008;283(46):32143-51.

108.   Khaminets A, Hunn JP, Könen-Waisman S, Zhao YO, Preukschat D, Coers J, et al. Coordinated loading of IRG resistance GTPases on to the *Toxoplasma gondii* parasitophorous vacuole. Cell Microbiol. 2010;12(7):939-61.

109.   Zhao YO, Khaminets A, Hunn JP, Howard JC. Disruption of the *Toxoplasma gondii* parasitophorous vacuole by IFN-γ-inducible immunity-related GTPases (IRG proteins) triggers necrotic cell death. PLoS Pathog. 2009;5(2):e1000288.

110.	Kravets E, Degrandi D, Ma Q, Peulen TO, Klumpers V, Felekyan S, et al. Guanylate binding proteins directly attack *Toxoplasma gondii* via supramolecular complexes. Elife. 2016;5.

111.	Konen-Waisman S, Howard JC. Cell-autonomous immunity to *Toxoplasma gondii* in mouse and man. Microbes Infect. 2007;9(14-15):1652-61.

112.	Fleckenstein MC, Reese ML, Konen-Waisman S, Boothroyd JC, Howard JC, Steinfeldt T. A *Toxoplasma gondii* pseudokinase inhibits host IRG resistance proteins. PLoS Biol. 2012;10(7):e1001358.

113.	Pawlowski N, Khaminets A, Hunn JP, Papic N, Schmidt A, Uthaiah RC, et al. The activation mechanism of Irga6, an interferon-inducible GTPase contributing to mouse resistance against *Toxoplasma gondii*. BMC Biol. 2011;9:7.

114.	Steinfeldt T, Konen-Waisman S, Tong L, Pawlowski N, Lamkemeyer T, Sibley LD, et al. Phosphorylation of mouse immunity-related GTPase (IRG) resistance proteins is an evasion strategy for virulent *Toxoplasma gondii*. PLoS Biol. 2010;8(12):e1000576.

115.	Murillo-Leon M, Muller UB, Zimmermann I, Singh S, Widdershooven P, Campos C, et al. Molecular mechanism for the control of virulent *Toxoplasma gondii* infections in wild-derived mice. Nat Commun. 2019;10(1):1233.

116.	Reese ML, Shah N, Boothroyd JC. The *Toxoplasma* pseudokinase ROP5 is an allosteric inhibitor of the immunity-related GTPases. J Biol Chem. 2014;289(40):27849-58.

117.	Reese ML. Immune to defeat. Elife. 2013;2:e01599.

118.	Afonso E, Thulliez P, Pontier D, Gilot-Fromont E. Toxoplasmosis in prey species and consequences for prevalence in feral cats: not all prey species are equal. Parasitology. 2007;134(Pt.14):1963-71.

119.	Guivier E, Galan M, Henttonen H, Cosson JF, Charbonnel N. Landscape features and helminth co-infection shape bank vole immunoheterogeneity, with consequences for Puumala virus epidemiology. Heredity (Edinb). 2014;112(3):274-81.

120.	Guivier E, Galan M, Salvador AR, Xuereb A, Chaval Y, Olsson GE, et al. Tnf-α expression and promoter sequences reflect the balance of tolerance/resistance to Puumala hantavirus infection in European bank vole populations. Infect Genet Evol. 2010;10(8):1208-17.

121.	Turner AK, Begon M, Jackson JA, Bradley JE, Paterson S. Genetic diversity in cytokines associated with immune variation and resistance to multiple pathogens in a natural rodent population. PLoS Genet. 2011;7(10):e1002343.

122.	Nikolin VM, Osterrieder K, von Messling V, Hofer H, Anderson D, Dubovi E, et al. Antagonistic pleiotropy and fitness trade-offs reveal specialist and generalist traits in strains of canine distemper virus. PLoS One. 2012;7(12):e50955.

123.	Bernstein-Hanley I, Coers J, Balsara ZR, Taylor GA, Starnbach MN, Dietrich WF. The p47 GTPases Igtp and Irgb10 map to the *Chlamydia trachomatis* susceptibility locus Ctrq-3 and mediate cellular resistance in mice. Proc Natl Acad Sci U S A. 2006;103(38):14092-7.

124.	Torelli F, Zander S, Ellerbrok H, Kochs G, Ulrich RG, Klotz C, et al. Recombinant IFN-γ from the bank vole *Myodes glareolus*: a novel tool for research on rodent reservoirs of zoonotic pathogens. Sci Rep. 2018;8(1):2797.

125.	Essbauer SS, Krautkramer E, Herzog S, Pfeffer M. A new permanent cell line derived from the bank vole (*Myodes glareolus*) as cell culture model for zoonotic viruses. Virol J. 2011;8:339.

126.	Singh U, Brewer JL, Boothroyd JC. Genetic analysis of tachyzoite to bradyzoite differentiation mutants in *Toxoplasma gondii* reveals a hierarchy of gene induction. Mol Microbiol. 2002;44(3):721-33.

127.   Fox BA, Falla A, Rommereim LM, Tomita T, Gigley JP, Mercier C, et al. Type II *Toxoplasma gondii* KU80 knockout strains enable functional analysis of genes required for cyst development and latent infection. Eukaryot Cell. 2011;10(9):1193-206.
128.   Altschul SF, Gish W, Miller W, Myers EW, Lipman DJ. Basic local alignment search tool. Journal of molecular biology. 1990;215(3):403-10.
129.   Song L, Florea L. Rcorrector: efficient and accurate error correction for Illumina RNA-seq reads. GigaScience. 2015;4:48.
130.   Grabherr MG, Haas BJ, Yassour M, Levin JZ, Thompson DA, Amit I, et al. Full-length transcriptome assembly from RNA-Seq data without a reference genome. Nat Biotec. 2011;29(7):644-52.
131.   Langmead B, Salzberg SL. Fast gapped-read alignment with Bowtie 2. Nat methods. 2012;9(4):357-9.
132.   Li H, Handsaker B, Wysoker A, Fennell T, Ruan J, Homer N, et al. The Sequence Alignment/Map format and SAMtools. Bioinformatics. 2009;25(16):2078-9.
133.   Simao FA, Waterhouse RM, Ioannidis P, Kriventseva EV, Zdobnov EM. BUSCO: assessing genome assembly and annotation completeness with single-copy orthologs. Bioinformatics. 2015;31(19):3210-2.
134.   Jackson JA, Begon M, Birtles R, Paterson S, Friberg IM, Hall A, et al. The analysis of immunological profiles in wild animals: a case study on immunodynamics in the field vole, *Microtus agrestis*. Mol Ecol. 2011;20(5):893-909.
135.   Zhang Y, Werling U, Edelmann W. Seamless Ligation Cloning Extract (SLiCE) cloning method. Methods Mol Biol. 2014;1116:235-44.
136.   Bernard P. Positive selection of recombinant DNA by CcdB. BioTechniques. 1996;21(2):320-3.
137.   Engler C, Marillonnet S. Golden Gate cloning. Methods Mol Biol. 2014;1116:119-31.
138.   Inoue H, Nojima H, Okayama H. High efficiency transformation of *Escherichia coli* with plasmids. Gene. 1990;96(1):23-8.
139.   Meerpohl HG, Lohmann-Matthes ML, Fischer H. Studies on the activation of mouse bone marrow-derived macrophages by the macrophage cytotoxicity factor (MCF). Eur J Immunol. 1976;6(3):213-7.
140.   Pluznik DH, Sachs L. The induction of clones of normal mast cells by a substance from conditioned medium. Exp Cell Res. 1966;43(3):553-63.
141.   lab Ws. L929 conditioned media preparation University of Calgary [Available from: https://winstonlab.ucalgary.ca/protocols/cultivation-1929-cells.]
142.   Khan M, Gasser S. Generating primary fibroblast cultures from mouse ear and tail tissues. JoVE. 2016(107).
143.   Amand MM, Hanover JA, Shiloach J. A comparison of strategies for immortalizing mouse embryonic fibroblasts. J Biol Met. 2016;3(2):41.
144.   Horisberger MA, de Staritzky K. A recombinant human interferon-αB/D hybrid with a broad host-range. J Gen Virol. 1987;68 (Pt 3):945-8.
145.   Berger Rentsch M, Zimmer G. A vesicular stomatitis virus replicon-based bioassay for the rapid and sensitive determination of multi-species type I interferon. PLoS One. 2011;6(10):e25858.
146.   Longo PA, Kavran JM, Kim MS, Leahy DJ. Transient mammalian cell transfection with polyethylenimine (PEI). Methods Enzymol. 2013;529:227-40.
147.   Hsu CY, Uludag H. A simple and rapid nonviral approach to efficiently transfect primary tissue-derived cells using polyethylenimine. Nat Protoc. 2012;7(5):935-45.
148.   Niewiadomski P, Rohatgi R. Rapid Screening of Gli2/3 Mutants Using the Flp-In System. Methods Mol Biol. 2015;1322:125-30.
149.   Chan FK, Moriwaki K, De Rosa MJ. Detection of necrosis by release of lactate dehydrogenase activity. Methods Mol Biol. 2013;979:65-70.

150. Niedelman W, Sprokholt JK, Clough B, Frickel EM, Saeij JP. Cell death of gamma interferon-stimulated human fibroblasts upon *Toxoplasma gondii* infection induces early parasite egress and limits parasite replication. IAI. 2013;81(12):4341-9.

151. Moudy R, Manning TJ, Beckers CJ. The loss of cytoplasmic potassium upon host cell breakdown triggers egress of *Toxoplasma gondii.* J Biol Chem. 2001;276(44):41492-501.

152. Hong HY, Yoo GS, Choi JK. Direct Blue 71 staining of proteins bound to blotting membranes. Electrophoresis. 2000;21(5):841-5.

153. Schafer H, Kliem G, Kropp B, Burger R. Monoclonal antibodies to guinea pig interferon-gamma: tools for cytokine detection and neutralization. J Immunol Methods. 2007;328(1-2):106-17.

154. Lilue J, Doran AG, Fiddes IT, Abrudan M, Armstrong J, Bennett R, et al. Sixteen diverse laboratory mouse reference genomes define strain-specific haplotypes and novel functional loci. Nat Genet. 2018;50(11):1574-83.

155. Schlegel M, Ali HS, Stieger N, Groschup MH, Wolf R, Ulrich RG. Molecular identification of small mammal species using novel cytochrome B gene-derived degenerated primers. Biochem Genet. 2012;50(5-6):440-7.

156. Farell EM, Alexandre G. Bovine serum albumin further enhances the effects of organic solvents on increased yield of polymerase chain reaction of GC-rich templates. BMC Research Notes. 2012;5(1):257.

157. Bienert S, Waterhouse A, de Beer TA, Tauriello G, Studer G, Bordoli L, et al. The SWISS-MODEL Repository-new features and functionality. Nucleic Acids Res. 2017;45(D1):D313-d9.

158. Pettersen EF, Goddard TD, Huang CC, Couch GS, Greenblatt DM, Meng EC, et al. UCSF Chimera--a visualization system for exploratory research and analysis. J Comput Chem. 2004;25(13):1605-12.

159. Szczesny RJ, Kowalska K, Klosowska-Kosicka K, Chlebowski A, Owczarek EP, Warkocki Z, et al. Versatile approach for functional analysis of human proteins and efficient stable cell line generation using FLP-mediated recombination system. PLoS One. 2018;13(3):e0194887.

160. Hausner J, Jordan M, Otten C, Marillonnet S, Buttner D. Modular Cloning of the Type III Secretion Gene Cluster from the Plant-Pathogenic Bacterium *Xanthomonas euvesicatoria*. ACS Synth Biol. 2019;8(3):532-47.

161. Fouriki A, Dobson J. Nanomagnetic Gene Transfection for Non-Viral Gene Delivery in NIH 3T3 Mouse Embryonic Fibroblasts. Materials. 2013;6(1):255-64.

162. Kawasaki H, Kosugi I, Arai Y, Iwashita T, Tsutsui Y. Mouse embryonic stem cells inhibit murine cytomegalovirus infection through a multi-step process. PLoS One. 2011;6(3):e17492.

163. Li J. Haplotypic polymorphism of the IRG protein family mediates resistance of mice against virulent strains of *Toxoplasma gondii*: Universität zu Köln; 2012.

164. Hermanns T, Muller UB, Konen-Waisman S, Howard JC, Steinfeldt T. The *Toxoplasma gondii* rhoptry protein ROP18 is an Irga6-specific kinase and regulated by the dense granule protein GRA7. Cell Microbiol. 2016;18(2):244-59.

165. Savan R, Ravichandran S, Collins JR, Sakai M, Young HA. Structural conservation of interferon gamma among vertebrates. Cytokine Growth Factor Rev. 2009;20(2):115-24.

166. Randal M, Kossiakoff AA. The structure and activity of a monomeric interferon-γ: α-chain receptor signaling complex. Structure. 2001;9(2):155-63.

167. Lapaque N, Takeuchi O, Corrales F, Akira S, Moriyon I, Howard JC, et al. Differential inductions of TNF-α and IGTP, IIGP by structurally diverse classic and non-classic lipopolysaccharides. Cell Microbiol. 2006;8(3):401-13.

168.	Gorissen M, de Vrieze E, Flik G, Huising MO. STAT genes display differential evolutionary rates that correlate with their roles in the endocrine and immune system. J Endocrinol. 2011;209(2):175-84.

169.	Parrini M, Meissl K, Ola MJ, Lederer T, Puga A, Wienerroither S, et al. The C-terminal transactivation domain of STAT1 has a gene-specific role in transactivation and cofactor recruitment. Front Immunol. 2018;9:2879.

170.	Stoltz M, Sundstrom KB, Hidmark A, Tolf C, Vene S, Ahlm C, et al. A model system for in vitro studies of bank vole borne viruses. PLoS One. 2011;6(12):e28992.

171.	Ramana CV, Gil MP, Han Y, Ransohoff RM, Schreiber RD, Stark GR. Stat1-independent regulation of gene expression in response to IFN-γ. Proc Natl Acad Sci U S A. 2001;98(12):6674-9.

172.	Chesler DA, Dodard C, Lee GY, Levy DE, Reiss CS. Interferon-γ-induced inhibition of neuronal vesicular stomatitis virus infection is STAT1 dependent. J Neurovirol. 2004;10(1):57-63.

173.	Voigt E, Inankur B, Baltes A, Yin J. A quantitative infection assay for human type I, II, and III interferon antiviral activities. Virol J. 2013;10:224.

174.	Hughes DJ, Kipar A, Leeming G, Sample JT, Stewart JP. Experimental infection of laboratory-bred bank voles (*Myodes glareolus*) with murid herpesvirus 4. Arch Virol. 2012;157(11):2207-12.

175.	Francois S, Vidick S, Sarlet M, Michaux J, Koteja P, Desmecht D, et al. Comparative study of murid gammaherpesvirus 4 infection in mice and in a natural host, bank voles. J Gen Virol. 2010;91(Pt 10):2553-63.

176.	Steed AL, Barton ES, Tibbetts SA, Popkin DL, Lutzke ML, Rochford R, et al. Gamma interferon blocks gammaherpesvirus reactivation from latency. J Virol. 2006;80(1):192-200.

177.	Hoffmann D, Franke A, Jenckel M, Tamosiunaite A, Schluckebier J, Granzow H, et al. Out of the reservoir: phenotypic and genotypic characterization of a novel Cowpox Virus isolated from a common vole. J Virol. 2015;89(21):10959-69.

178.	Tsai CY, Hu Z, Zhang W, Usherwood EJ. Strain-dependent requirement for IFN-γ for respiratory control and immunotherapy in murine gammaherpesvirus infection. Viral Immunol. 2011;24(4):273-80.

179.	Seeber F, Boothroyd JC. Escherichia coli β-galactosidase as an in vitro and in vivo reporter enzyme and stable transfection marker in the intracellular protozoan parasite *Toxoplasma gondii*. Gene. 1996;169(1):39-45.

180.	Murray PJ. Macrophages as a battleground for toxoplasma pathogenesis. Cell Host Microbe. 2011;9(6):445-7.

181.	Sharma L, Wu W, Dholakiya SL, Gorasiya S, Wu J, Sitapara R, et al. Assessment of phagocytic activity of cultured macrophages using fluorescence microscopy and flow cytometry. Methods Mol Biol. 2014;1172:137-45.

182.	Takács AC, Swierzy IJ, Lüder CGK. Interferon-γ restricts *Toxoplasma gondii* development in murine skeletal muscle cells via nitric oxide production and Immunity-Related GTPases. PLoS One. 2012;7(9):e45440.

183.	Herrmann DC, Pantchev N, Vrhovec MG, Barutzki D, Wilking H, Frohlich A, et al. Atypical *Toxoplasma gondii* genotypes identified in oocysts shed by cats in Germany. Int J Parasitol. 2010;40(3):285-92.

184.	Polley L. Navigating parasite webs and parasite flow: emerging and re-emerging parasitic zoonoses of wildlife origin. Int J Parasitol. 2005;35(11-12):1279-94.

185.	Karesh WB, Dobson A, Lloyd-Smith JO, Lubroth J, Dixon MA, Bennett M, et al. Ecology of zoonoses: natural and unnatural histories. Lancet. 2012;380(9857):1936-45.

186.	Han BA, Schmidt JP, Bowden SE, Drake JM. Rodent reservoirs of future zoonotic diseases. Proc Natl Acad Sci U S A. 2015;112(22):7039-44.

187.   Kołodziej-Sobocińska M. Factors affecting the spread of parasites in populations of wild European terrestrial mammals. Mammal Research. 2019.
188.   Maizels RM, Nussey DH. Into the wild: digging at immunology's evolutionary roots. Nat Immunol. 2013;14(9):879-83.
189.   Jackson JA. Immunology in wild nonmodel rodents: an ecological context for studies of health and disease. Parasite Immunol. 2015;37(5):220-32.
190.   Turner AK, Paterson S. Wild rodents as a model to discover genes and pathways underlying natural variation in infectious disease susceptibility. Parasite Immunol. 2013;35(11):386-95.
191.   Shwab EK, Saraf P, Zhu XQ, Zhou DH, McFerrin BM, Ajzenberg D, et al. Human impact on the diversity and virulence of the ubiquitous zoonotic parasite *Toxoplasma gondii*. Proc Natl Acad Sci U S A. 2018;115(29):E6956-E63.
192.   Galal L, Schares G, Stragier C, Vignoles P, Brouat C, Cuny T, et al. Diversity of *Toxoplasma gondii* strains shaped by commensal communities of small mammals. Int J Parasitol. 2019;49(3-4):267-75.
193.   Yang H, Wang JR, Didion JP, Buus RJ, Bell TA, Welsh CE, et al. Subspecific origin and haplotype diversity in the laboratory mouse. Nat Genet. 2011;43(7):648-55.
194.   Schlotterer C, Tobler R, Kofler R, Nolte V. Sequencing pools of individuals - mining genome-wide polymorphism data without big funding. Nat Rev Genet. 2014;15(11):749-63.
195.   Migalska M, Sebastian A, Radwan J. Profiling of the TCRβ repertoire in non-model species using high-throughput sequencing. Sci Rep. 2018;8(1):11613.
196.   Kloch A, Babik W, Bajer A, Sinski E, Radwan J. Effects of an MHC-DRB genotype and allele number on the load of gut parasites in the bank vole *Myodes glareolus*. Mol Ecol. 2010;19 Suppl 1:255-65.
197.   Gazzinelli RT, Mendonca-Neto R, Lilue J, Howard J, Sher A. Innate resistance against *Toxoplasma gondii*: an evolutionary tale of mice, cats, and men. Cell Host Microbe. 2014;15(2):132-8.
198.   Rohfritsch A, Galan M, Gautier M, Gharbi K, Olsson G, Gschloessl B, et al. Preliminary insights into the genetics of bank vole tolerance to Puumala hantavirus in Sweden. Ecol Evol. 2018;8(22):11273-92.
199.   Szücs I. Polymorphism in non-coding region affects expression of the innate immune defense gene IFIH1 in the bank vole (*Myodes glareolus*). [Bachelor Degree Project]. In press 2018.
200.   Melo MB, Nguyen QP, Cordeiro C, Hassan MA, Yang N, McKell R, et al. Transcriptional analysis of murine macrophages infected with different *Toxoplasma* strains identifies novel regulation of host signaling pathways. PLoS Pathog. 2013;9(12):e1003779.
201.   Jang H, Abraham SJ, Chavan TS, Hitchinson B, Khavrutskii L, Tarasova NI, et al. Mechanisms of membrane binding of small GTPase K-Ras4B farnesylated hypervariable region. J Biol Chem. 2015;290(15):9465-77.
202.   Jackson JA, Hall AJ, Friberg IM, Ralli C, Lowe A, Zawadzka M, et al. An immunological marker of tolerance to infection in wild rodents. PLoS Biol. 2014;12(7):e1001901.
203.   Ohshima J, Sasai M, Liu J, Yamashita K, Ma JS, Lee Y, et al. RabGDIalpha is a negative regulator of interferon-γ-inducible GTPase-dependent cell-autonomous immunity to *Toxoplasma gondii*. Proc Natl Acad Sci U S A. 2015;112(33):E4581-90.
204.   Khan A, Behnke MS, Dunay IR, White MW, Sibley LD. Phenotypic and gene expression changes among clonal type I strains of *Toxoplasma gondii*. Eukaryot Cell. 2009;8(12):1828-36.

205.   Yang N, Farrell A, Niedelman W, Melo M, Lu D, Julien L, et al. Genetic basis for phenotypic differences between different *Toxoplasma gondii* type I strains. BMC genomics. 2013;14:467.

206.   Liu Y, Mi Y, Mueller T, Kreibich S, Williams EG, Van Drogen A, et al. Multi-omic measurements of heterogeneity in HeLa cells across laboratories. Nat Biotech. 2019;37(3):314-22.

207.   Dastagir K, Reimers K, Lazaridis A, Jahn S, Maurer V, Strauss S, et al. Murine embryonic fibroblast cell lines differentiate into three mesenchymal lineages to different extents: new models to investigate differentiation processes. Cell Reprogram. 2014;16(4):241-52.

208.   Sharma R, Parker S, Al-Adhami B, Bachand N, Jenkins E. Comparison of tissues (heart vs. brain) and serological tests (MAT, ELISA and IFAT) for detection of *Toxoplasma gondii* in naturally infected wolverines (*Gulo gulo*) from the Yukon, Canada. Food Waterborne Parasitol. 2019:e00046.

209.   Dubey JP, Frenkel JK. Toxoplasmosis of rats: a review, with considerations of their value as an animal model and their possible role in epidemiology. Vet Parasitol. 1998;77(1):1-32.

210.   Gotteland C, Chaval Y, Villena I, Galan M, Geers R, Aubert D, et al. Species or local environment, what determines the infection of rodents by *Toxoplasma gondii?* Parasitology. 2014;141(2):259-68.

211.   Bastien M, Vaniscotte A, Combes B, Umhang G, Germain E, Gouley V, et al. High density of fox and cat faeces in kitchen gardens and resulting rodent exposure to *Echinococcus multilocularis* and *Toxoplasma gondii.* Folia Parasitol. 2018;65.

212.   Dumetre A, Darde ML. How to detect *Toxoplasma gondii* oocysts in environmental samples? FEMS microbiology reviews. 2003;27(5):651-61.

213.   Schares G, Vrhovec MG, Pantchev N, Herrmann DC, Conraths FJ. Occurrence of *Toxoplasma gondii* and *Hammondia hammondi* oocysts in the faeces of cats from Germany and other European countries. Vet Parasitol. 2008;152(1-2):34-45.

214.   Waap H, Vilares A, Rebelo E, Gomes S, Angelo H. Epidemiological and genetic characterization of *Toxoplasma gondii* in urban pigeons from the area of Lisbon (Portugal). Vet Parasitol. 2008;157(3-4):306-9.

215.   Montoya A, Miro G, Mateo M, Ramirez C, Fuentes I. Molecular characterization of *Toxoplasma gondii* isolates from cats in Spain. J Parasitol. 2008;94(5):1044-6.

216.   Fuentes I, Rubio JM, Ramirez C, Alvar J. Genotypic characterization of *Toxoplasma gondii* strains associated with human toxoplasmosis in Spain: direct analysis from clinical samples. J Clin Microbiol. 2001;39(4):1566-70.

217.   Yan X, Ji Y, Liu X, Suo X. Nitric oxide stimulates early egress of *Toxoplasma gondii* tachyzoites from human foreskin fibroblast cells. Parasit Vectors. 2015;8:420.

218.   Tomita T, Yamada T, Weiss LM, Orlofsky A. Externally triggered egress is the major fate of *Toxoplasma gondii* during acute infection. J Immunol. 2009;183(10):6667-80.

219.   Matta SK, Patten K, Wang Q, Kim BH, MacMicking JD, Sibley LD. NADPH oxidase and Guanylate Binding Protein 5 restrict survival of avirulent Type III strains of *Toxoplasma gondii* in naive macrophages. MBio. 2018;9(4).

220.   Jokelainen P, Nylund M. Acute fatal toxoplasmosis in three Eurasian red squirrels (*Sciurus vulgaris*) caused by genotype II of *Toxoplasma gondii*. J Wildl Dis. 2012;48(2):454-7.

221.   Virreira Winter S, Niedelman W, Jensen KD, Rosowski EE, Julien L, Spooner E, et al. Determinants of GBP recruitment to *Toxoplasma gondii* vacuoles and the parasitic factors that control it. PLoS One. 2011;6(9):e24434.

222.   Kim CY, Zhang X, Witola WH. Small GTPase Immunity-Associated Proteins mediate resistance to *Toxoplasma gondii* infection in Lewis rat. IAI 2018;86(4).

223.   Dubey JP, Ferreira LR, Alsaad M, Verma SK, Alves DA, Holland GN, et al. Experimental Toxoplasmosis in rats induced orally with eleven strains of *Toxoplasma gondii* of seven genotypes: tissue tropism, tissue cyst size, neural lesions, tissue cyst rupture without reactivation, and ocular lesions. PLoS One. 2016;11(5):e0156255.
224.   Cirelli KM, Gorfu G, Hassan MA, Printz M, Crown D, Leppla SH, et al. Inflammasome sensor NLRP1 controls rat macrophage susceptibility to *Toxoplasma gondii*. PLoS Pathog. 2014;10(3):e1003927.
225.   Cavailles P, Flori P, Papapietro O, Bisanz C, Lagrange D, Pilloux L, et al. A highly conserved Toxo1 haplotype directs resistance to toxoplasmosis and its associated caspase-1 dependent killing of parasite and host macrophage. PLoS Pathog. 2014;10(4):e1004005.
226.   Cavailles P, Sergent V, Bisanz C, Papapietro O, Colacios C, Mas M, et al. The rat Toxo1 locus directs toxoplasmosis outcome and controls parasite proliferation and spreading by macrophage-dependent mechanisms. Proc Natl Acad Sci U S A. 2006;103(3):744-9.
227.   Gorfu G, Cirelli KM, Melo MB, Mayer-Barber K, Crown D, Koller BH, et al. Dual role for inflammasome sensors NLRP1 and NLRP3 in murine resistance to *Toxoplasma gondii*. MBio. 2014;5(1).
228.   Ewald SE, Chavarria-Smith J, Boothroyd JC. NLRP1 is an inflammasome sensor for *Toxoplasma gondii*. IAI. 2014;82(1):460-8.
229.   Witola WH, Mui E, Hargrave A, Liu S, Hypolite M, Montpetit A, et al. NALP1 influences susceptibility to human congenital toxoplasmosis, proinflammatory cytokine response, and fate of *Toxoplasma gondii*-infected monocytic cells. IAI. 2011;79(2):756-66.
230.   Witola WH, Liu SR, Montpetit A, Welti R, Hypolite M, Roth M, et al. ALOX12 in human toxoplasmosis. IAI. 2014;82(7):2670-9.
231.   Kim BH, Chee JD, Bradfield CJ, Park ES, Kumar P, MacMicking JD. Interferon-induced guanylate-binding proteins in inflammasome activation and host defense. Nat Immunol. 2016;17(5):481-9.
232.   Zimmerman LM, Bowden RM, Vogel LA, Tschirren B. A vertebrate cytokine primer for eco-immunologists. Funct Ecol. 2014;28(5):1061-73.
233.   Arakawa T, Alton NK, Hsu YR. Preparation and characterization of recombinant DNA-derived human interferon-γ. J Biol Chem. 1985;260(27):14435-9.
234.   Arakawa T, Hsu YR, Narachi MA, Herrera C, Rohde MF, Hennigan P. Reversibility of acid denaturation of recombinant interferon-γ. Biopolymers. 1990;29(6-7):1065-8.
235.   Kendrick BS, Cleland JL, Lam X, Nguyen T, Randolph TW, Manning MC, et al. Aggregation of recombinant human interferon gamma: kinetics and structural transitions. J Pharm Sci. 1998;87(9):1069-76.
236.   Tobler SA, Fernandez EJ. Structural features of interferon-gamma aggregation revealed by hydrogen exchange. Protein Sci. 2002;11(6):1340-52.
237.   Sugimura K, Higashi N. A novel outer-membrane-associated protease in *Escherichia coli*. J Bacteriol. 1988;170(8):3650-4.
238.   Sugimura K, Nishihara T. Purification, characterization, and primary structure of Escherichia coli protease VII with specificity for paired basic residues: identity of protease VII and OmpT. J Bacteriol. 1988;170(12):5625-32.
239.   Slodowski O, Bohm J, Schone B, Otto B. Carboxy-terminal truncated rhuIFN-γ with a substitution of Gln133 or Ser132 to leucine leads to higher biological activity than in the wild type. Eur J Biochem. 1991;202(3):1133-40.
240.   Nacheva G, Todorova K, Boyanova M, Berzal-Herranz A, Karshikoff A, Ivanov I. Human interferon gamma: significance of the C-terminal flexible domain for its biological activity. Arch Biochem Biophys. 2003;413(1):91-8.

241.   Lundell D, Lunn C, Dalgarno D, Fossetta J, Greenberg R, Reim R, et al. The carboxyl-terminal region of human interferon gamma is important for biological activity: mutagenic and NMR analysis. Protein Eng. 1991;4(3):335-41.

242.   Döbeli H, Gentz R, Jucker W, Garotta G, Hartmann DW, Hochuli E. Role of the carboxy-terminal sequence on the biological activity of human immune interferon (IFN-γ). J Biotech. 1988;7:199-216.

243.   Dufour A, Bellac CL, Eckhard U, Solis N, Klein T, Kappelhoff R, et al. C-terminal truncation of IFN-γ inhibits proinflammatory macrophage responses and is deficient in autoimmune disease. Nat Comm. 2018;9(1).

244.   Tolkacz K, Bednarska M, Alsarraf M, Dwuznik D, Grzybek M, Welc-Faleciak R, et al. Prevalence, genetic identity and vertical transmission of *Babesia microti* in three naturally infected species of vole, *Microtus* spp. (Cricetidae). Parasit Vectors. 2017;10(1):66.

245.   Vannier EG, Diuk-Wasser MA, Ben Mamoun C, Krause PJ. Babesiosis. Infect Dis Clin North Am. 2015;29(2):357-70.

246.   Aguilar-Delfin I, Homer MJ, Wettstein PJ, Persing DH. Innate resistance to *Babesia* infection is influenced by genetic background and gender. IAI. 2001;69(12):7955-8.

247.   Clawson ML, Paciorkowski N, Rajan TV, La Vake C, Pope C, La Vake M, et al. Cellular immunity, but not gamma interferon, is essential for resolution of *Babesia microti* infection in BALB/c mice. IAI. 2002;70(9):5304-6.

248.   Igarashi I, Suzuki R, Waki S, Tagawa Y, Seng S, Tum S, et al. Roles of CD4(+) T cells and gamma interferon in protective immunity against *Babesia microti* infection in mice. IAI. 1999;67(8):4143-8.

249.   Droescher M, Begitt A, Marg A, Zacharias M, Vinkemeier U. Cytokine-induced paracrystals prolong the activity of signal transducers and activators of transcription (STAT) and provide a model for the regulation of protein solubility by small ubiquitin-like modifier (SUMO). J Biol Chem. 2011;286(21):18731-46.

250.   Anderson SE, Jr., Remington JS. Effect of normal and activated human macrophages on *Toxoplasma gondii*. J Exp Med. 1974;139(5):1154-74.

251.   Most J, Spotl L, Mayr G, Gasser A, Sarti A, Dierich MP. Formation of multinucleated giant cells in vitro is dependent on the stage of monocyte to macrophage maturation. Blood. 1997;89(2):662-71.

252.   Dupont SA, Goelz S, Goyal J, Green M. Mechanisms for regulation of cellular responsiveness to human IFN-beta1a. J Interferon Cytokine Res. 2002;22(4):491-501.

253.   Liang X, Shin YC, Means RE, Jung JU. Inhibition of interferon-mediated antiviral activity by murine gammaherpesvirus 68 latency-associated M2 protein. J Virol. 2004;78(22):12416-27.

254.   Trilling M, Le VT, Zimmermann A, Ludwig H, Pfeffer K, Sutter G, et al. Gamma interferon-induced interferon regulatory factor 1-dependent antiviral response inhibits vaccinia virus replication in mouse but not human fibroblasts. J Virol. 2009;83(8):3684-95.

255.   Decker T, Kovarik P, Meinke A. GAS elements: a few nucleotides with a major impact on cytokine-induced gene expression. J Interferon Cytokine Res. 1997;17(3):121-34.

256.   Axtner J, Sommer S. Validation of internal reference genes for quantitative real-time PCR in a non-model organism, the yellow-necked mouse, *Apodemus flavicollis*. BMC Res Notes. 2009;2:264.

257.   Rueda-Martinez C, Fernandez MC, Soto-Navarrete MT, Jimenez-Navarro M, Duran AC, Fernandez B. Identification of reference genes for Quantitative Real Time PCR assays in aortic tissue of Syrian hamsters with bicuspid aortic valve. PLoS One. 2016;11(10):e0164070.

258.   Brown AJ, Gibson S, Hatton D, James DC. Transcriptome-based identification of the optimal reference CHO genes for normalisation of qPCR Data. Biotechnol J. 2018;13(1).

259.   Babik W, Stuglik M, Qi W, Kuenzli M, Kuduk K, Koteja P, et al. Heart transcriptome of the bank vole (*Myodes glareolus*): towards understanding the evolutionary variation in metabolic rate. BMC genomics. 2010;11:390.

260.   Migalska M, Sebastian A, Konczal M, Kotlik P, Radwan J. De novo transcriptome assembly facilitates characterisation of fast-evolving gene families, MHC class I in the bank vole (*Myodes glareolus*). Heredity (Edinb). 2017;118(4):348-57.

261.   Suwinska A, Tarkowski AK, Ciemerych MA. Pluripotency of bank vole embryonic cells depends on FGF2 and activin A signaling pathways. Int J Dev Biol. 2010;54(1):113-24.

10. Publikationsverzeichnis

1. Ferreira S. C. M.*, **Torelli F.***, Klein S., Fyumagwa R., Karesh W. B., Hofer H., Seeber F., East M. L. (2019). Evidence of high exposure to *Toxoplasma gondii* in free-ranging and captive African carnivores. *Int J Parasitol: Parasites Wildl.* **8,** 111–117 (2019) (* shared first authorship)

2. **Torelli F.**, Zander S., Ellerbrok H., Kochs G., Ulrich R. G., Klotz C., Seeber F., Recombinant IFN-γ from the bank vole *Myodes glareolus*: a novel tool for research on rodent reservoirs of zoonotic pathogens. *Sci. Rep.* **8,** 2797 (2018)

3. Ehret T., **Torelli F.**, Klotz C., Pedersen A. B., Seeber F. Translational rodent models for research on parasitic protozoa – a review of confounders and possibilities. *Front. Cell. Infect. Microbiol.* **7,** 238 (2017)

4. Gibellini L., Pinti M., Beretti F., Pierri C.L., Onofrio A., Riccio M., Carnevale G., De Biasi S., Nasi M., **Torelli F.**, Boraldi F., De Pol A., Cossarizza A., Sirt3 interacts with Lon protease and regulates its acetylation status. *Mitochondrion* **18,** 76–81 (2014)

11. Funding sources

Funded by the Research Training Group 2046 "Parasite Infections: From Experimental Models to Natural Systems" funded by the Deutsche Forschungsgemeinschaft (DFG, German Research Foundation) and the Agnes und Georg Blumenthal-Stiftung.

12. Selbständigkeitserklärung

Hiermit bestätige ich, dass ich die vorliegende Arbeit selbständig angefertigt habe. Ich versichere, dass ich ausschließlich die angegebenen Quellen und Hilfen in Anspruch genommen habe.

Ort   Datum   Unterschrift